After Everybody Else Gave Up

Dignity 'n Retirement

JOE PRIEST

PAGE PUBLISHING, INC.
New York, NY

First originally published by Page Publishing, Inc. 2017

ISBN 978-1-68409-452-3 (Paperback)
ISBN 978-1-68409-453-0 (Digital)

Photo and Image Credits
Robinson, Dee. NCAA Baseball Photos
http://tarletonbaseball.smugmug.com

Baseball Image Credits to Cox, Rebecca

Printed in the United States of America

In baseball, behind 8-0 in the late innings can stir up a tide of frustration. One single event can add a spark to start a rally. In the bottom of the seventh inning, seven singles and two more hits was enough to ignite one of the most inspiring comebacks in World Series history. Whether on the world stage as these 1929 Philadelphia Athletics or in an exercise lab in the kinesiology building, coming back from an apparently hopeless situation is thrilling and timeless.

Contents

Preface

No longer is it questionable that exercise is beneficial to health and well-being; it is now acknowledged in "Exercise is Medicine™" (American College of Sports Medicine, 2009). The American College of Sports Medicine (ACSM), the American Medical Association (AMA), and many others are calling on all physicians and health-care workers to make physical activity and exercise a standard part of a disease prevention and treatment medical paradigm in the United States (Sallis, 2009). *After Everybody Else Gave Up* is written for the literally millions of individuals and families who have "fallen through the cracks" of the health care or disease care system, many of whom have lost hope. In the words of many of our individuals in training, they have typically been told by the system that there is "nothing else we can do." Conventional exercise facilities are ill-equipped to deliver effective exercise training to these individuals who have depleted their insurance coverage (if they had any) and lost their jobs and their independence. My book tells the story of the Laboratory for Wellness and Motor Behavior, a remarkably effective university training program that provides no-cost supervised exercise programs for individuals with spinal cord injuries, cerebral palsy, stroke, spina bifida, muscular dystrophy, multiple sclerosis, Guillain Barrè syndrome, and other neuromuscular disabilities.

The story is told in chapters (1) from my perspective as the professor who developed the program, (2) from the trainers who manage the rehabilitation, (3) from the individuals and families who have nowhere else to go for help, (4) from fellow university faculty, (5) from a hospital administrator, and (6) from a key physician. The book was purposefully written as an easy read—like a conversation you might have in the bleachers at a Sunday afternoon baseball game. For some who do not choose to read the book cover to cover, the "Players" subchapters include, for convenience, some repetitive information on trainers or equipment and direct the reader to a name and particular disability of interest. The stories contributed freely by the so-called clients provide real insight into the challenges encountered in attaining and regaining wellness. These subchapters provide details of individuals who are improving wellness and motor behavior *after everybody else gave up.*

Acknowledgments

Without the support of numerous Kinesiology Department Chairpersons, the progress of this unique lab would have been impossible. My thanks go to Drs. Joe Gillespie, Wendell Sadler, Steve Crews, Kayla Peak, and Steve Simpson, across more than twenty years of lab operations. Special thanks also goes to Russell Jennings, who developed the Psycle and the OrthoSys (IntelliGEN, Wichita Falls, TX), which enabled us to provide rehabilitation services at the university. My gratitude is extended to the hundreds of clients and students who worked cooperatively through difficult times when progress was slow and doubt crept in. Special thanks go to doctoral student and former NCAA baseball player Andy Wolfe for bringing his energy, enthusiasm, and love of the game to the Department of Kinesiology. His passion and wit was infectious. Finally, I would like to thank the late Dr. R. Donald Hagan, my mentor, my friend, and the former Director of Exercise Physiology at the Johnson Space Center, for his collaboration, support, and encouragement to the Laboratory for Wellness and Motor Behavior.

Introduction

Retirees in America are large in number and diversity. For the purposes of this book, the subgroups include three general retiree audiences: individuals who currently have limited access to the labor market. These individuals are involuntarily retired because of various physical disabilities, such as spinal cord injury, cerebrovascular accident (stroke), spina bifida, cerebral palsy, multiple sclerosis, Guillain-Barrè syndrome, and numerous other neuromuscular, joint, or skeletal issues; those who are approaching retirement from the labor force—a relatively large group. We are on the precipice of the greatest retirement crisis in the history of the world (see Siedel, 2013); and people who are currently retired—a disproportionate number in relation to the active labor force.

The US Census released 2015 statistics identifying an estimated 46.2 million people older than sixty-five years (see Millennials Outnumber Baby Boomers, 2015). As retirees leave the workforce, the direct and indirect impact is significant. From the individual perspective, adjusting to this new lifestyle, many opportunities and limitations are realized. During this critical adjustment period, habitual behavior may have a big impact on health outcomes. There is little dignity in loss of health. This book attempts to present the positive and negative prospects after retirement.

The focus is on the trainers and the individuals engaged in supervised training in the Laboratory for Wellness and Motor Behavior (LWMB), a facility in the Department of Kinesiology at Tarleton State University, a part of the Texas A&M University System. The LWMB, with some imagination has the operational characteristics of a baseball team: owner, general manager, coaches, players, clubhouse, grounds crew, training and game facilities, and a competitive schedule. Often-used phrases from the game of baseball symbolize some of the challenges, adjustments, personal interactions, accomplishments, victories, and defeats encountered in this unique lab.

A key role in program operation is served by graduate and undergraduate students who volunteer for a three-hundred-hour internship in the LWMB, which fulfills a departmental requirement for an Applied Learning Experience. These special students are profiled here in order to describe to the reader just who they are and how they respond to their training responsibilities. Selected representatives are described to the reader with details obtained from personal interviews and blog posts.

The volunteer clients are typically dismissed from conventional health care (everybody else gave up). Faculty and pre-professional students in the LWMB design and closely supervise physical activity programs for each individual. The program operates with the similar budget of other physical activity classes at the University Department of Kinesiology. The program is offered, with no fees required, to individuals after they obtain releases for physical training from their physicians. The stories presented here represent the prospect of maintaining/improving wellness and motor behavior after retirement.

Most of these clients have left the workforce involuntarily. Individuals introduced in this manuscript will provide stories of people who experienced transformative changes in their lives due to disease or disability. They openly share their stories of loss of independence through disease or injury, their rehabilitation efforts, the perceived abandonment of conventional care, and often their loss of hope for recovery. Their stories are real, and each person unselfishly shares his/her experiences, responses, coping behaviors, bouts with depression, and motivations that help them face another day with hope.

The purpose of this book is to stimulate hope for recovery in millions of individuals and impacted family members; it is purposefully written as simplistic, practical, and relatable, like it might be told from the ball park on a sunny spring day. It sheds light on and offers a solution to the growing problems encountered with the expanding retiree populations. Our team at the LWMB stands ready to replicate the program across the country and around the world.

What's the Problem?

The health of Americans is under careful watch. We now have quick Internet access to (1) rankings and research, (2) best hospitals, (3) doctor finder, (4) best health plans, (5) best Medicare plans, (6) best nursing homes, (7) best diets, and (8) top recommended health products. In 2013, the audience was over 20 million unique visitors with 120 million page views (see *U.S. News and World Report*, 2015). Years ago, the World Health Organization (WHO) identified the problem of lack of physical activity, stating that it could be among the ten leading causes of death and disability in the world while also pointing out that it is, for the most part, entirely preventable. They reported that "sedentary lifestyles increase all causes of mortality, double the risk of cardiovascular diseases, diabetes and obesity, and increase the risks of colon cancer, high blood pressure, osteoporosis, lipid disorders, depression and anxiety" ("Physical Inactivity a Leading Cause of Disease and Disability" 2002).

With all this available information, a significant disconnection becomes obvious when we visit with the consumers represented by the clients in the LWMB. In each of their cases, they obtained necessary medical care and were prescribed conventional therapy and perhaps some in-home or institutional therapy. Then in a few weeks, they got released from care, coincidentally, with the end of insurance coverage. This is understandable but not reasonable. Orthopedic injuries from sports or other accidents may respond favorably to six weeks of physical therapy, whereas a staggering number of other more serious injuries need much-extended attention, even years with continuing assistance for recovery.

After retirement from the labor force, job placement may be difficult at best and probably impossible for those who retired involuntarily because of disease or injury. At fifty dollars or more per hour, continued professional assistance becomes unattainable. This book describes the experiences

and interpretations of these released clients and pre-professional trainers, their responses to a low-stress, no-cost university training program, which was made indefinitely available.

Involuntary Retirement

Stroke. Of the involuntarily retired, about seven million
people are alive today after surviving a stroke. There are two
forms of stroke: *ischemic*—blockage of blood vessels supply-
ing the brain, and *hemorrhagic*—bleeding into or around the
brain (Office of Communications and Public Liaison [NIH]
2004). Over 80 percent of all strokes are ischemic, commonly
caused by blood clots that interrupt the blood flow in an area
of the brain. Most do not know about or do not receive the
clot-busting drug tPA, which has to be administered within
three hours of the beginning of the stroke symptoms. Strokes
occur in more than 795,000 Americans, killing almost 130,000
each year, and cost the US an estimated $34 billion (Centers
for Disease Control and Prevention 2015). Cerebrovascular

accidents (strokes) often cause unilateral paralysis; however, subsequent joint problems secondary to the stroke compound the difficulty of rehabilitation.

The first state of rehabilitation usually begins twenty-four to forty-eight hours after a stroke, followed by physical therapy, a home caregiver, and often a skilled nursing facility. Medicines are used to treat memory loss, insomnia, pain, anxiety, future blood clotting, and depression (WebMD 2015), sometimes all together (my observations in the LWMB). One study reported the annual costs of outpatient rehabilitation services and medicine for a stroke survivor was over seventeen thousand dollars (Godwin 2011). Conventional therapy rarely lasts for more than about six weeks or until the insurance money is depleted. Some conventional treatments may place the paralyzed limb in a sling or brace. This is sufficient stimulus to cause the limb to adapt to being immobile, contributing to subsequent contractures and stiff or frozen joints of the hip, knee, ankle, shoulder, elbow, wrist, and fingers.

The National Stroke Association (NSA) has as its mission to reduce the incidence and impact of stroke by developing education and programs focused on prevention, treatment, rehabilitation and support for all impacted by stroke. In 2014, over $3.3 million was spent on management, fundraising, and stroke education. For over thirty years, the search continues for more effective and creative ways to manage this devastating problem (Hope After Stroke 2016).

Spinal cord injuries (SCI) affect between four and five million Americans per year. There are about three hundred thousand people in the United States living with spinal cord injuries. Most spinal cord injuries occur between the ages of sixteen and thirty years, and about 79 percent of those who experience spinal cord injuries are male (see BrainandSpinalCord.org 2015). The average annual health care and living expenses that are directly attributable to SCI vary with the severity of the injury. The two rodeo cowboys highlighted in this book are classified as low tetraplegics (C6-C7 injuries) and might incur the average annual expenses of $111,237. Other SCI individuals have injuries that resulted in paraplegia, and members of this group incur a reported average annual expense of $67,415 (DeVivo 2011).

Life expectancy of persons with SCI has improved considerably thus contributing to the increased risk of secondary health conditions, which include pressure sores, urinary and respiratory tract infections, osteoporosis, obesity, diabetes, and cardiovascular disease. These conditions each contribute to reduced quality of life. Efforts are ongoing to develop effective interventions to enhance active lifestyles and fitness, thus preventing some of the secondary problems (van der Woude and ALLRISC 2013).

Since 1973, the American Spinal Injury Association (ASIA) has been serving members and medical professionals in the search for optimal care, education, and research. The Reeve Foundation has invested approximately $110 million on research to develop effective treatments for acute and spinal cord injury, most of which was spent on the infrastructure and delivery of therapy. Approximately 88 percent of all SCI individuals are released from conventional care to private homes (Christopher & Dana Reeve Foundation 2016).

Cerebral palsy (CP) is the most common of all childhood disabilities. About 764,000 individuals, including 500,000 children under the age of eighteen years currently have CP (see

CerebralPalsy.org 2015). In one study among children enrolled in Medicaid in 2005, medical costs were ten times higher than for children without CP ($16,721 vs. $1674 in 2005 dollars) (Centers for Disease Control and Prevention 2015).

Training programs for CP include systematic efforts to increase muscle strength. Most of the studies conducted from 1966 through 2000 demonstrated strength increases with no negative side effects. One systematic review of strength training in this population found improvements in activity and improvement in self-perception (Dodd 2002). No single standard training protocol exists. Individual differences in people with CP require careful evaluation, and planned activities should be tailored to the individual needs (Harvey 2008).

United Cerebral Palsy (UCP) affiliates provide services and support to ensure life without limits. The group works to advance the independence, productivity, and full citizenship of people with disabilities. In 2013, the group spent over $2.9 million dollars on affiliate support, public policy analysis/advocacy, public education, and non-federal grants (Life Without Limits for People with Disabilities 2015).

The best estimate of the incidence of multiple sclerosis (MS) in the U.S. is about 400,000 people with an estimated 2.3 million diagnosed worldwide (National Multiple Sclerosis Society 2015). A recent estimate of average direct and indirect expenses associated with MS ranged from $8,528 to $54,244 per patient per year, where prescription drugs accounted for the majority of the direct costs (Adelman 2013).

A quick and common Internet search for "Treatments for Multiple Sclerosis" finds first many drug options and reference to the benefits of exercise. "One to three sessions may be enough… to assess symptoms, see how well you can handle different tasks, and show you exercises you can do at home" (Mellen Center for Multiple Sclerosis, Cleveland Clinic 2014). Suggestions on living and thriving with MS include managing muscle strength, range of motion, and stretching.

The National Multiple Sclerosis Society (NMSS) raises awareness by building connections and engaging people in addressing the current challenges of MS while moving toward long-term solutions for tomorrow. They invested over two million dollars in professional education and training and fourteen million in public education for the year ending September 30, 2014 (Raise Awareness 2016).

Individuals with spina bifida present impairments in muscle and sensory functions of lower limbs related to the level of spinal involvement, resulting in restrictions in activities of daily living. Benefits of physical activities and training are still under investigation (Ivanyi 2014). Bracing is often used to aid mobility (Mazur 2004); however, possible adverse effects related to long-term use of bracing are not well-established. Walking with the aid of forearm crutches may have favorable effects compared to walking without crutches (Vankoski 1997).

Although fetal surgical treatments are evolving, the management of adults is still uncertain. Suggested physical activity programs should be tailored for the individual and should be varied, fun, and rewarding. Much like able-bodied individuals, exercise should be moderate-intensity exercise for 150 minutes per week, including two or more days per week of strength training (UAB/Lakeshore Research Collaboration 2015).

The Spina Bifida Association (SBA) actively raises awareness about spina bifida. Through a process of education, its volunteers work together to improve the outlook of over 177,000 Americans who live with the challenges of spina bifida each day. In 2014, program services included over $1.3 million, including over $.5 million dedicated to education (Educators: Health Information Sheets 2015).

Orthopedic disorders affect the body's musculoskeletal system and include arthritis, bursitis, fibromyalgia, low-back pain, carpal tunnel syndrome, and other painful joint problems that may take the individual out of the work force. Arthritis alone affects 52.5 million US adults—it is the most common cause of disability (Center for Disease Control and Prevention 2014).

Most office visits to orthopedic surgeons are injury related and often related to the knee, back, and shoulder. According to the National Center for Health Statistics (NCHS), the visit rate increased with age groups forty-five to sixty-four years old and did not increase with age up to 75 years (Centers for Disease Control and Prevention 1998). The Arthritis Foundation (AF) publishes *Arthritis Today* that reaches 4.2 million readers with life-changing information and resources as well as guidelines to access optimal care (Athritis Foundation 2016).

Our search for solutions to attaining and maintaining dignity after involuntary retirement continues through these concentrated national efforts. The personnel and financial commitment outlined above is stunning and the need for new resources is eminent.

Approaching Retirement

In the decades to come, we will witness millions of elderly Americans, the baby boomers and others, slipping into poor health and poverty. Too frail to work and too poor to retire, they will become the new normal for many elderly Americans (Siedel 2013). In 2011, the first of the baby-boom generation reached retirement age, and for the next eighteen years, boomers will be turning sixty-five at a rate of about eight thousand people per day (Alyne Ellis 2011).

Currently Retired

As people leave the labor force, they often leave an active routine and replace it with more inactivity. The rigors of a job, some physical, some emotional, or social, encourage movement and engagement with others. Much of this activity is *eustress*, or beneficial stress which people handle effectively. Some activity becomes *distress* and difficult to manage, even if not perceived by the individual. Survivors of the work force learn to cope, at least, and perhaps conquer the different degrees of stress. After leaving the work force, for whatever reason, new stressors are encountered; some of those are unexpected. After years of labor, more available leisure time with less money can be stressful as the retiree spends more time off the clock. This is true for volunteer retirees but even more critical for individuals who leave the labor force because of an inability to maintain employment.

Factors

The Editor-in-Chief of *Popular Science* suggested in the July 2015 periodical, "Dare to Dream Big." Even speaking of technology, the phrase seems applicable to the search for solutions to the incomplete rehabilitation of life-changing disabilities and injuries. The journal editor Ransom suggests this approach has the "ability to bring a brighter day" (2015). Our own Dr. Neal, in his second season at the LWMB, submitted that on the front door should be "Hope Begins Here" (Sutherland 2015). Coming from our own actively-participating physician, this carries special meaning for our continued efforts toward complete rehabilitation and return to active lifestyle.

Dr. Lewis Thomas acknowledges that problems exist in the American health-care system, but not everything is bad, and perhaps we should be celebrating "our general good shape." Years ago, he noted that life expectancy continues to increase, we are beginning to make progress in our understanding of chronic diseases and that sooner or later, we will learn to cope effectively with most of these. We will still age away and die, but the aging, and even the dying, can become a healthy process. Furthermore,

when a healthy old creature dies, there is no outside evil force, nor any central flaw. The dying is built into the system so that it can occur at once, at the end of a pre-clocked, genetically determined allotment of living. Centralization ceases, the forces that used to hold cells together are disrupted, the cells lose recognition of each other, chemical signaling between cells comes to an end, vessels become plugged by thrombi and disrupt their walls, bacteria are allowed free access to tissues normally forbidden, organelles inside cells begin to break apart; nothing holds together; it is the bursting of billions of bubbles, all at once. (Thomas 1979)

Dr. Thomas credits inspiration for this view to Dr. Oliver Wendell Holmes in his 1858 poem entitled "The One-Hoss Shay," as in Thomas' book source "The Deacon, symbolizing Nature, who designs the perfect organism. He designed a perfect chaise, in his imagination, without a weak spot so it couldn't break down. In his timeless poem:

the weakest part mus' stan' the strain;

'N' the way t' fix it, uz I maintain,

Is only jest

T' make that place uz strong uz the rest.

There was respectable, decent, proper sort of aging of the chaise after one hundred years. Then at the hour of death:

the wheels were just as strong as the thills,

And the floor was just as strong as the sills,

And the panels just as strong as the floor...

And the back crossbar as strong as the fore...

And yet, as a whole, it is past a doubt

In another hour it will be worn out!

Dr. Thomas describes Dr. Holmes's death scene: "No tears, no complaints, no listening closely for last words. No brief. Just, in the way of the world, total fulfillment."

All at once the horse stood still,

Close by the meet'n'-house on the hill

All at once the horse stood still

First a shiver, and then a thrill,

Then something decidedly like a spill,

And the parson was sitting upon a rock,

At half-past nine by the meet'n'-house clock....

What do you think the parson found,

When he got up and stared around?

The poor old chaise in a heap or mound,

As if it had been to the mill and ground!

You see, of course, if you're not a dunce,

How it went to pieces all at once,

All at once, and nothing first,

Just as bubbles do when they burst

(Holmes 1858)

We spend a lot of money on individuals after retirement, much of it offset by government assistance. A recent government report (*The State of Aging and Health in America, 2013*) stated that more than 25% of all Americans and 67 percent of older Americans have multiple chronic conditions, and treatment for this population accounts for 66 percent of the country's health care budget. Much of this expense prolongs patient misery rather than improving quality of life (Bell 2013). In 2004, it was reported that 30 percent of all Medicare expenditures are attributed to the 5 percent of beneficiaries that die each year, with one-third of that cost occurring in the last month of life (Banarto 2004). More of these funds might be directed at a plan, as Holmes envisioned, to mobilize all we know about building the perfect organism without a weak spot so it couldn't break down.

The ability to move around effectively and safely is fundamental to the health and our well-being, perhaps more so for older adults. "When you are thankful and grateful for what you're doing in life, even when you are spread thin, it helps immediately with giving you the energy and motivation to get things done," says Larry Marks, a clinical psychologist at the University of Central Florida (Gold 2014). Prolonged access to physical activity throughout retirement may diminish, or even reverse, the deleterious effects of sedentary living (D. S. Willoughby et al.; 2000; Blankenship and Priest 2000; D. S. Willoughby et al. 2002; Simpson and Priest 2005) and help moderate the disproportionate health-care expense now experienced in the different groups of retirees. Movement includes walking for leisure and daily activities, exercising, driving a car, or transferring from a bed to a chair.

Limitations can lead to dependence and other adverse outcomes, including increased risk for cardiovascular disease, cancer, injuries secondary to falls, automobile crashes, and depression (National Center for Chronic Disease Prevention and Health Promotion 2013). "Staying active and social prolongs life even after age 75," says Miriam E. Nelson, director of Tufts' John Hancock Research Center on Physical Activity, Nutrition, and Obesity Prevention. The benefit of exercise is not linear across the fitness spectrum; "The biggest jump comes at the very bottom of the range. The less active you are now, the more benefit you get from adding even a small amount of exercise to your life" (2012).

Depression is the leading cause of disability worldwide, according to the World Health Organization (WHO). New strategies for treating the illness are desperately needed. A sense of social isolation is a key factor in its development. Group associations exert powerful psychological effects because humans are social beings, and interacting with others is vital to our well-being. Joining one or more groups is a cost-effective treatment and can both prevent and cure depression. Although family relationships are the most protective, association with a different type of family may be similarly effective, more so than association with individuals. The type of group is not important as long as it matters to the individual (Cruwys 2014).

Rizzuto and colleagues from the Karolinska Institute followed 1810 men and women age seventy-five years and up for eighteen years. They reported that, among other life-style factors, maintaining a rich social network was almost as important as exercise ("Lifestyle, Social Factors, and Survival After Age 75: Population Based Study," 2012). Greg Anderson suggests that the triumphant patient lives life, despite all the troubles, in a celebration of the moment, and we make the future an extension of these moments of wellness. Bernie S. Siegel, MD, the author of *Love, Medicine, and Miracles* writes in the introduction for Anderson's book, *The Triumphant Patient* (2001), that the book inspires, instructs, gives hope, and it heals. In the face of pain and debilitating deterioration, he offers a choice to focus the mind on principles of wellness rather than on factors of dying. Where there is hope, there is life; moreover, there is hope in any situation.

In my Human Performance Laboratory for the past twenty years, I had a passion for improving the wellness of individuals who had various degrees of paralysis. Some had chronic disease, some had injuries, but what became apparent was that it was difficult/impossible for them to access the benefits of exercise. The first ten years, we investigated the benefits of movement on paralyzed muscle tissue, collaborating with fellow faculty, mentoring students, and utilizing limited available resources. The results were peer-reviewed and systematically presented at consecutive annual national conferences of the American College of Sports Medicine. As a professor, I observed that the experience was constructive for my students who frequently were challenged with the presentation on the national stage. I used to say, "Not rocket science," but that became curiously contradictory when my own mentor and co-author, the late Dr. Don Hagan, became Director of Exercise Physiology at the Johnson Space Center.

Robert Priest, kinship acknowledged, was diagnosed with prostate cancer, which he faced with Nancy, his wife of fifty years. As a public school teacher and an administrator, they had maintained very active lifestyles while helping raise two boys and later three grand-daughters and three grand-sons. Following the diagnosis, together they moved four hundred miles to the city of the treatment facility where he endured forty-four proton beam treatments over a nine-week period. After returning home for a few weeks, he was diagnosed with a paranasal carcinoma, which was promptly treated with radiation, complete with destructive side-effects. Robert and Nancy used their faith and found hope in recovery only to meet another challenge in four-vessel coronary artery disease, severe enough that surgical stents were not possible. Following the life-saving and traumatic coronary artery bypass surgery, Robert said with his all-American smile, he identified possible additions to his BS and his University of Texas MS degrees—WCS to indicate that when things went wrong, they were each Worse Case Scenarios. With this triumphant spirit, he looks forward to age ninety-five.

The preceding description of Robert is as it was after the first draft writing of this manuscript. Including the original story serves to emphasize how our situation may change in a heartbeat as in Robert's case, when a blood clot lodged in the brain. The WCS got even worse. At breakfast one day, he had trouble stirring his morning cup of coffee; his right side "just did not feel right." That was the early signs of a stroke that he mistakenly attributed to the preceding day's hard work in his shop. What followed were three consecutive clots over two days, causing much brain damage. He lost movement on his dominant right side as well as his ability to swallow (aphagia) and had difficulty speaking (dysphasia). After five days in critical care, surgeons implanted a gastric feeding tube in order to get nutrients into his stomach.

Robert's stroke just became a factor; it made my laboratory experience most meaningful. The problems related to training paralyzed muscles just got very personal and like in crisis situations, I can think of little else except helping to restore health to my brother. After conventional rehabilitation, he was released before recovery of wellness and motor behavior. Fifteen currently training stroke survivors in our university LWMB demonstrated the *esprit de corps* by sending collective encouragement to Robert. The feelings of pride, fellowship, and common loyalty are shared by the members of this unique group. He and Nancy moved 250 miles to gain access to major league recovery. Like James Earl Jones' *Field of Dreams* character, professional writer Terrence Mann said when he chose to follow the ghost team into the corn field, "If I have the courage to follow through with this… what a story it will make."

Evolving Approaches

The idea for exercise therapies for people with disabilities came in the late 1800s. Dr. R. Tate McKenzie contributed a medical article, "The Therapeutic Uses of Exercise" (1894), advocating the aspects of exercise that made it therapeutic:

> It relieves congestion by equalizing circulation... acts as a sedative to the nervous system probably through its action on the circulation, strengthens and enlarges muscle, bones, and ligaments, and would thus apply to all conditions caused by weakness or inequality of development. (McKenzie, 566)

Between 1904 and the beginning of the First World War, Dr. McKenzie lectured and practiced medicine, and he wrote two volumes of his book *Exercise in Education and Medicine* (1909), which made contributions to physical education, public health, and physical therapy. Dr. McKenzie is credited with the first instance of adaptive physical education to aid the overall development as human beings. His concluding chapter of the 1909 book was "The Treatment of Locomotor Ataxia by Exercise," and he credits Swiss physician H. S. Frenkel (The Treatment of Tabetic Ataxia by Means of Systematic Exercises 1902) with developing a therapy that "took patients through a graduated series of exercises, with the aim of progressive muscular control." Treating paralytic polio, he recommended "rest and support of the limb in the acute stage, then voluntary movement, electricity, and massage to keep up the muscle tone… vibration… and re-educational movements performed before a mirror…" (McKenzie 1909, 550–551). During that time period, "this combination treatment was fairly typical, as physicians struggled to cope with… a disease they did not really understand until well into the twentieth century" (Rogers 1996).

During World War I between 1915 and 1918, McKenzie expanded his concept of exercise to include passive movement and electrical stimulation to aid in the maintenance and development of muscle tone and nerve sensitivity. The rehabilitation improved not only his future civil life, it also decreased the financial impact on the individual and the nation (Treatment of Convalescent Soldiers by Physical Means 1917; Reclaiming the Maimed at War 1918). Later McKenzie compiled his wartime writings into a booklet entitled *Reclaiming the Maimed: A Handbook of Physical Therapy*, which provided the basis of modern physical medicine (1918). Few individuals have made such significant contributions as McKenzie. An exhaustive 2008 review of his efforts is contributed by Fred Mason ("R. Tate McKenzie's Medical Work and Early Exercise Therapies for People with Disabilities" 2008).

Senior living communities are developed to offer senior adults and retirees a full continuum of care. These communities are common facilities where peer support is encouraged and maximized to extend independence. Typically located minutes from shopping centers, restaurants, hospitals, and other conveniences, transportation may be offered to reach destinations. Some facilities include comprehensive packages including chef-prepared meals, daily activity calendars, pools, managers, and month-to-month leases. Social, learning, and spiritual activities provide a wide array of possibilities to optimize the living experience. As the importance of physical activity becomes more and more recognized, access to daily group exercise classes may be available. All of these conveniences are made available at considerable expense—a quick survey revealed available leases from $2,150 to $4,950 and more per month. These living communities may satisfy the needs of many retirees who are prepared to pay the price.

Throughout the country, senior village programs plan communities for homeowners at least fifty-five years of age, which included over 39.5 million households. By 2020, *U.S. News and World Report* suggested that 45 percent of American households will be headed by someone who is over fifty-five years old. This arrangement allows for seniors to stay in their own homes and might be looked at as a way "to cost-effectively serve a graying nation." In Madison, Wisconsin, a program called "Supporting Active Independent Lives" or SAIL, a pharmacist and university pharmacy students provide personal health coaching to its members. Older adults are often overmedicated; more than 1,500 seniors are hospitalized each year because of adverse side events, according to SAIL Executive Director Ann Albert (Moeller 2011). Excellent summary information is available in the *State of Aging & Health in America 2013* (Centers for Disease Control and Prevention 2015).

Impaired mobility is associated with a variety of adverse health outcomes. By creating unique integrated interventions across disciplines, we can improve mobility and health for older Americans. Dr. Ron Savage, president of the Sarah Jane Brain Foundation reported that the effects of therapy are improved health and ambulation (getting out of wheelchairs more) through aided walking and biking. If we strengthen these neural pathways that are working, they will end up connecting with other neural pathways (International Brain Injury Association, 2013). Donald O. Hebb, a Canadian psychologist, summarized a memory theory that would come to dominate the field. He suggested that "neurons that fire together wire together" (Skaggs 2014).

Tegan Cruwys and Genevieve Dingle are lecturers and clinical psychologists at the University of Queensland in Australia. Along with their colleague S. Alexander Haslam, a social psychologist and advisor for *Scientific American Mind*, reports that joining groups is a cost-effective, stand-alone treatment strategy in the absence of traditional therapy, even calling it the social cure. Important group relations exert powerful psychological effects because humans are social beings. Groups provide a sense of belonging, giving life meaning, something that is lost in depression.

Herb Benson, a Harvard MD has spent more than thirty years investigating at length the power of the mind to change the body's response to stress. Earlier terms used to describe the mind/body connection included the placebo effect that elicits our innate capacity for self-healing. Benson introduced the Relaxation Response, observing that the effect was unlike the placebo effect, which is neither predictable nor reproducible. People got better simply because they imagined themselves better. Dr. Benson suggested that "the immense, trans-forming power of the mind and body, of our beliefs, and of self-perpetuated healing will remain within us—eternally."

Thirty-five years ago, when I was a young cardiolo-gist, I noticed a trend among my patients with high blood pressure, or hypertension, a silent and dan-gerous precursor of heart disease. Once I prescribed medications, I noticed they often complained about fainting or becoming dizzy. These were side effects of having their blood pressures lowered with med-ications. Patients went from feeling fine to being burdened with irritating and disabling side effects, all the result of medicine I had prescribed. (Benson 1975)

These ideas were implemented at the Benson-Henry Institute for Mind Body Medicine in 2006 at the Massachusetts General Hospital where an initial study reported that their program reduced the participants' medical visits by 43 percent in the year after taking part. The lead investigator Dr. James E. Stahl suggested that the mind-body approach "promotes wellness… and could potentially ease the burden on our health delivery systems at minimal cost and at no real risk" (Relaxation Response and Resiliency Training and Its Effect on Healtcare Resource Utilization 2015).

Another advocate of the mind and body approach is expressed by another Harvard physician Dr. Jeffrey Rediger. Also a Princeton-trained theologian, he interpreted in a December 2015 TED talk the difference between our Western and Eastern culture.

The brilliance of Western culture lies in its capacity to recognize distinctions and analyze the parts of the larger hole. In Eastern framework, however, there is no such sharp distinction… In Eastern medicine both physical and mental illnesses are treated by rebalancing the body's energetic system.

Dr. Rediger spoke of two colleagues who were both diagnosed by biopsy with terminal cancers—no known treatments. Years later, both had CTs that read negative for cancer. Is it possible that the mind played a role in the recovery? He has spent his professional career clarifying this relationship. "There are powers in your heart and your mind that no medicine can touch." Obtained from interviews of individuals who have overcome hopeless diseases, Rediger states "Every person I have spoken with has affected a deep change in perception of themselves in the world." Furthermore, "The interface of the body, mind and the soul may well be the most profound mystery of our time" ("A Medicine of Hope and Possibility" 2015).

The contribution of the mind to the health of the body is long recognized and undeniable. Malcomb Gladwell in his book *Blink* (*Blink: The Power of Thinking Without Thinking* 2005) reported how we think without thinking. Dean Ornish, MD, in Martin Rossman's book *Guided Imagery for Self-Healing* (2000) points out that your mind and your body communicate in images, and this imagery can be used for healing.

This so-called Guided Imagery uses attention, intention and imagination to create desirable changes in the body. The first basic research between the body, brain, and central nervous system was termed psychoneuroimmunology. William H. Foege (Public Health and Preventive Medicine 1985) suggested that:

> the most important determinants of health and longevity will be the personal choices made by each individual… changes in our behavior—both external and internal—can reduce the large number of premature deaths and illnesses and lead to better health and longer life.

Valerie Harper, fighting cancer that was supposed to be terminal in three months, found hope at age seventy-five in her battle in what they say about "the three pillars of health: nutrition, exercise, and naps" (Grant, Meg 2015, Feb/Mar, 14–17). Modern technology, including PET (positron electron tomography) scans and NMR (nuclear magnetic resonance) imaging contribute to our understanding of how and why imagery affects healing.

Working in a professional position at the Cooper Institute for Aerobics Research for Dr. Kenneth Cooper (the Father of Aerobics), Dr. Marius Maianu's position on exercise comes as no surprise:

> By keeping up with the recommended minimum amount of aerobic exercise per week (150 minutes of moderate intensity exercise per week), you can significantly lower your risk of death due to a cardiac event. Research also shows that there's no real benefit to ranking in the 'superior' category of risk factors. The greatest benefit and reduction in risk factors is in making it from 'very poor' or 'poor' to at least 'fair,' and it doesn't take much to get there... It's just a matter of moving. (Maianu 2015)

In summary, early recognition of the necessity to be physically active to the creation of focus societies, to the evolution of senior communities and senior villages, and to help in affecting a positive change in clients' perceptions of themselves, the LWMB's game plan for wellness appears to be working. The rehabilitation game in the conventional health-care system has become skewed in in the middle or later innings. A lifetime of funds are being spent on the acute medical care and a few weeks of a short-term contract in physical therapy, leaving nothing in the later innings.

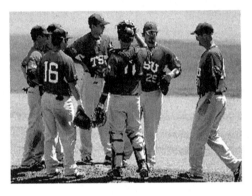

In baseball, it is like multiple meetings on the pitcher's mound, rotating all the team's pitchers through in one tough inning, leaving the bullpen decimated. You spend the final innings with your fourth reliever's 80–mph fastballs delivered over the middle of the plate getting hammered. You've got the wrong guy on the mound, and your game plan is in shambles.

Risks/Benefits

Physical inactivity is identified as a leading contributor to premature mortality (Hallal 2012). Approximately 25–35 percent of American adults are living sedentary lives, exposing them to the hazard of inactivity, including health problems and even early death. Steven Blair is a professor of exercise science and epidemiology at the University of South Carolina's Arnold School of Public Health. Speaking at the American Psychological Association Annual Convention, he called American's physical inactivity "the biggest problem health problem of the twenty-first century." A man who is even moderately active and fit has only half the risk of developing numerous health conditions and lives six years longer than an unfit man. Habitual exercise also delays the mind's decline and is good for brain health overall.

Blair added, "We need numerous changes to promote more physical activity for all, including public policies, changes in the health care system, promoting activity in educational settings and worksites, and social and physical environmental changes" (American Psychological Association 2009).

For years, it has been recognized that participation in physical activity is complicated and influenced by many factors, including "demographic, biological, cognitive, emotional, sociocultural, and environmental factors" (Bauman 2002). Accordingly, the barriers to adopting a physically active lifestyle are equally complex although the health benefits are no longer deniable. The absolute risk of complications from physical exertion is very low. Of the approximately six hundred thousand annual deaths from heart disease, only a small fraction is exercise-related.

In the 2009 edition of American College of Sports Medicine's *Exercise is Medicine: A Clinician's Guide to Exercise Prescription* (2009), it was suggested that the pre-screen for exercise should answer the question: "Is this patient safe to remain sedentary?" In June 2014, the American College of

Sports Medicine (ACSM) convened a scientific roundtable to establish best practices in the exercise pre-participation health screening process. One of the concerns was that the recommended screening process often eliminates the very individuals who would benefit the most from exercise. Their simplified version of the exercise screen recommended approval from health-care providers for medical clearance to engage in exercise. This decision should be made "on the basis of the presence of signs or symptoms and/or known cardiovascular, metabolic, or renal disease and physical activity status" (Riebe 2015).

Physically inactive but otherwise healthy asymptomatic persons may begin light- to moderate-intensity exercise without medical clearance (Garber 2011) and, in the absence of symptoms, progress gradually in intensity as recommended by ACSM exercise prescription guidelines (American College of Sports Medicine 2014). These simplified health screening criteria serve to provide more people access to the benefits of exercise. Further rationale for our low-intensity, high-volume approach to training individuals who have physical limitations comes from the summary statement: "The greatest health benefits emerge when a person alters a sedentary lifestyle and becomes just moderately physically active" (McArdle 2007). In addressing the needs of diverse populations, exercise professionals must be able to adapt exercise to meet the unique needs, concerns, and abilities of each individual. The consensus is that for a great majority of individuals, the benefits of regular exercise far outweighs the risks. Physicians are thus increasingly agreeable to prescribing exercise in our LWMB for their patients.

In the LWMB, we accept the challenge of preparing student-interns for a future that we do not even yet comprehend. It is unpredictable yet we recognize their extraordinary capacities for innovation. There is risk involved in empowering student-interns as they create unique training activities for clients. Robinson suggests that we are educating people out of their creative capacities. Creativity is as important in education as literacy, and we should treat it with the same status. Students should not be frightened of being wrong. If they are not prepared for imperfection, they will never come up with anything original ("Do Schools Kill Creativity?" 2006). He adds in a subsequent TED talk that the real role of leadership in educational is to create a climate of possibility. We have to "engage [students], their curiosity, their individuality, and their creativity. That's how you get them to learn" ("How to Escape Education's Death Valley" 2013). Robinson himself is a master of engaging the learner as his invited talks have been viewed on the TED website over thirty-six million times (2006).

Awareness of the problem of being a couch potato is beginning to peak with retirees as indicated by the availability of a new Health Care Costs Calculator (Love, Robert, ed. 2015, Feb/Mar), allowing the user to estimate expenses related to 10 extra pounds, use of tobacco, and lack of exercise. The loss of health, wealth, and happiness is real. These problems encountered in retirement may seem overbearing at times and prompt the idea of "calling the game on account of darkness."

Even being currently recognized as a pinch hitter in rehabilitation efforts, the improvements in wellness and motor behavior recorded in our lab suggest that the benefits are far-reaching. Not only do the clients improve, but the unique experience of the trainers may be an education beyond the college curriculum. The LWMB supervised exercise program may well be the difference between winning and losing. It probably looks surprising as an unlikely solution to attaining the goal of "Dignity 'n Retirement." After all, as our critics say from the foul line, "It's just exercise."

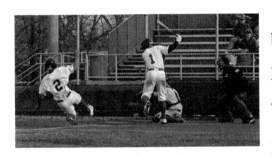

It's similar in baseball to stealing home. It looks simple. The element of surprise is significant. It is very rare and best accomplished when strategically communicated and executed by the coach, third-base runner, and the right-handed batter. The steal has to be well orchestrated, the base runner getting an early jump during the wind up by the pitcher, the batter holding his ground in the batter's box shielding the catcher's view of the base runner, and finally the base runner arriving at home plate and sliding under the catcher's tag. The high risk is recognized, but the reward may be the difference in the outcome of the game.

Clubhouse—Sets of 1000

The clubhouse is our training facility which is approximately one thousand six hundred square feet of floor space housing various pieces of equipment selected to accommodate people who have exercise limitations. The mission of the LWMB is to provide access to the benefits of exercise to those who are currently excluded from the health care system. Being unlike any other training facility, we use our over achievers [my designation] in the Department of Kinesiology and other departments on special arrangement to deliver exercise services to students and other clients who have various neuromuscular diseases and disabilities. These individuals have typically been dismissed from medical and therapeutic care, often because of the lack of or the termination of insurance coverage. For those individuals, the prospect of attaining or regaining wellness restores hope. This may look to them like a place where dreams come true.

Training in the LWMB is basically in a community environment. Formulation of our approach to training was partly digital, obtained from earlier studies (Priest 1996; Ferguson and Priest 2000; Gardner and Priest 2002; Balkenbush and Priest 2003; Balkenbush 2005), and partly evidential from twenty years of training experience. Based upon other investigations of passive training of paralyzed muscles (McKenzie, R., 1918; Willoughby D. S., 2000; 2002), our training regimen includes low-intensity, high-volume repetitions using the entire body, including paralyzed limbs. The delivery of the exercise prescription is more of an art than a science. Because no two people are alike, day-to-day and even minute-to-minute feedback from clients allows for continual modifications of the activities. We are much like a card, domino, poker, or coffee club, but our game is supervised exercise. The social interaction between and among clients and student-interns is encouraged and practiced daily not because of a written protocol but because the trainer volunteer recognizes the impor-tance of a genuine interest in the client as a person.

Animal scientist and autism advocate Temple Grandin, who personally revamped the animal welfare and food safety industry, said, "We've got to get people connected to real, physical stuff—it teaches problem solving (On How to Raise Resilient Animals 2015). For the student intern, get-ting them connected in this Applied Learning Experience has been highly valued by those who completed three hundred hours of service in the LWMB[1]. Student-interns are providing continuous attention to each client while they are in the lab. Student-interns are not passing out workouts or studying on their phones, clipboards, or somebody else's written exercise protocols; they are attending to clients. At the time of writ-ing this, forty-three individuals were actively participating in supervised training. For example, although we were training fourteen stroke survivors, each one is unique and responds to attention and training differently. Every day is a new challenge

---

[1] See selected comments/posts at the Google+ Community called "Stroke Rehab" at https://plus.google.com/u/0/commu nities/112013677417890656684.

to respond to their present condition or state of health and state of mind, which may change very slowly or sometimes rapidly. We are a service facility—our product is the predictable benefit that results from extensive rhythmic movement of the entire body, including paralyzed limbs. Depending upon the individual case, the client may begin workouts on the T5 NuStep (NuStep, Inc., Ann Arbor, Michigan) with easy gliding motions then gravitate to the OrthoSYS Dynamic Weight-bearing System (IntelliGEN, Wichita Falls, Texas) then to conventional parallel bars then to the Psycle (direct-drive, energy-regeneration, recumbent leg cycle ergometer, IntelliGEN, Wichita Falls, Texas). Other appropriate equipment used in symmetrical training includes the Excite TOP, an upper-body ergometer (UBE) made by Technogym, USA Corporation (Fairfield, New Jersey). Although there is not one protocol to improve the wellness and motor behavior of our clients, all of these activities cause bilateral training stimulus—that is, both sides of the body experience similar movements.

Bilateral training is critical in preparation for gait training. Other conventional training facilities may attempt walking and strive for greater distances, even in a walker, before the core or pelvis is stable. For instance, following a stroke and resulting weakness or paralysis on one side, premature walking attempts will employ such an abnormal gait that training may actually cause more problems. Poor body alignment often causes lower back pain that may become debilitating—a result, not of the injury or disease but of the training. This awful scenario may then worsen and include drug prescriptions to combat the back pain.

In the LWMB, after perhaps months of preparation for walking, clients may gravitate from bilateral training to ambulation with a walker, cane, or student intern. Irene, whom you will meet later, graduated from her wheel chair after months of the previously described bilateral training to walking in what she called her hovering position. She walked unassisted with her hand just over the hand or shoulder of the student-intern within the confines of the training room. As her gait and her confidence improved, trainers expanded her path outside the clubhouse.

The kinesiology building includes gymnasia, offices, and classrooms bordered by a wide hallway. The resulting pathway is nearly a square and about 440 feet (134.1 m) long, often, in the spirit of our training team referred to as our base path. The distance between the bases is one hundred ten feet, and the resulting diamond is just strides away from the LWMB clubhouse.

The LWMB recognizes the value of community, what we do we do together in the spirit of a team. In my high school, the Olton Mustangs coaches taught us to break the team huddles with "all for one and one for all." Memories of this routine conjure up the pride and commitment we felt as players, and I now recognize how profound that was—it still resonates half a century later in the LWMB. During laboratory activities, we train side by side, we talk to each other, we continually celebrate accomplishments, and we confide in each other—a common consensual sharing agreement. We recognize, as Yogi observed, "Ninety percent of the game is half mental."

Leadership in the LWMB is based upon an educational philosophy taken from Albert Einstein's address on October 15, 1936, ("Out of My Later Years" 1950) on the occasion of the three hundredth anniversary of higher education in America; it states that "the school should always have as its aim the development of a harmonious personality... The development of general ability for independent thinking and judgment should always be placed at the forefront, rather than the acquisition of special knowledge." To this end, the LWMB intern/trainers are given extensive liberty in the selection of the material to be taught and the methods of teaching employed by them. The motive for work in the LWMB "is the pleasure in work, pleasure in its result, and the knowledge of the value of the result to the community." Einstein continues that "the hands of service must ever be at work... and to these serving hands mine also shall belong" (1950).

Einstein (1950) stated that "the most important method of education... always has consisted of that in which the pupil was urged to actual performance...," and he credits an unnamed source who defined education in this way:

"Education is that which remains, if one has forgotten every-thing he learned in school." It is with this approach that the LWMB attempts to provide a hands-on learning experience for students that will be remembered long after graduation.

Most of my professorial responsibilities are for teaching; therefore, the trainers often make important independent decisions based upon their understanding of basic training principles. Professional publication and presentation of activ-ities in the LWMB has been ongoing since 1994. These stu-dent-led reports were peer-reviewed and accepted for presen-tations at state and national conferences.

This university-based supervised exercise program is delivered to individuals with various disabilities, includ-ing spinal injury, strokes, multiple sclerosis, cerebral palsy, Guillain-Barrè syndrome, spina bifida, and others with neu-romuscular problems who otherwise are left unserved by current practices. The diligence with which these individuals approach training is nothing short of inspiring. In 2015, they collectively completed over seven thousand workouts under our supervision. On the newly added NuStep equipment in ten months, the group completed nearly three million arm and leg steps recorded just on those two devices. This provides obvious evidence that clients will take advantage of this training opportunity.

The lab is directed by faculty and managed by pre-professional students and offered as an Applied Learning Experience to disabled students at the university then conditionally to individuals in the community and surrounding geographic area. Bridging the gap between technology, escalating medical costs, and deteriorating health in aging, the LWMB attempts to bring "science and the everyday experience of human beings… together in meaningful ways," a phrase borrowed from Dr. Herbert Benson in describing the emergence of mind/body medicine.

The administrative organization of the LWMB was patterned after the method used by Abraham Lincoln informally inspecting the Union Army troops in the early part of the American Civil War, later termed "management by wandering around." Walmart founder, Sam Walton, was also famous for getting in behind the scenes to see how the business was working. He rode in delivery trucks in order to better understand any problems encountered from that angle. He liked to "get away from all the noise about the latest management framework or the next idea about how leadership should be done." He treated employees as associates of the business, encouraging and facilitating their investments in the business. An admitted non-conformist, he said, "I have always been driven to buck the system, to innovate, to take things beyond where they've been" (Bergdahl 2006).

On the front door of the LWMB, among other things, is the phrase "question convention—encourage invention," which promotes, as Walton suggested, innovation and solving problems as they arise. In the absence of strategic treatment protocols for individuals with severe disabilities, the training activities are individualized, even among folks with similar challenges. No two stroke survivors are alike; some have lost the ability to speak (aphasia), some have difficulty speaking (dysphasia), while others have no trouble with language but rather with cognition. Many experience paralysis on one side (hemiplegia) to various degrees. Even after release from medical care and conventional therapy, some still have partial or even total loss of muscle function in one leg, arm, hand, and fingers. Similarly for other disabilities that are too soon dropped from health care, the LWMB offers a concerned, friendly, and informed approach to improving the health and wellness to all who are willing and able to take advantage of this exercise approach.

This simplistic idea motivates our game. It inspires the no-cost, no-time-limit, continuous, high-repetition-movement community regimen that is employed by the LWMB. We intend to add a spark that starts a rally in every individual. Continued innovation and ongoing results of these hands-on training efforts will contribute to future facility and program design that will optimize the health of retirees.

The General Managers— Trainers in the LWMB

Who are the student/leaders in the LWMB? They are scholars first; they have successfully completed the general education requirements for language, math, science, speech, social studies, history, political science, and creative arts. The final two years of the degree focus on their chosen field of study and include kinesiology, exercise physiology, motor behavior, strength and conditioning, prevention and care of injuries, first aid, and adaptive, corrective, and developmental exercise. In addition, as a major in kinesiology, each student must demonstrate gender and age-adjusted fitness in cardiovascular health, flexibility, and body composition. They choose to complete their requirements for the bachelor's degree in kinesiology by volunteering to work under a faculty mentor in a hands-on, unpaid internship. During this semester, they have many Applied Learning Experiences with hands-on opportunities as a pre-professional to screen, assess, prescribe, and supervise exercise programs aimed at improving the overall wellness and movement skills of individuals representing various populations.

The student-interns here after a fairly typical educational process of sixteen to eighteen years are themselves recovering from prolonged and necessary focus on their own success. In their final semester, the internship affords them an opportunity to learn selflessness, to be more considerate of others than themselves. Most with excellent levels of health and fitness required for the degree in kinesiology, they learn sometimes for the first time to communicate with individuals who have compromised health and fitness. The training teams in the LWMB are empowered to create and administer adaptive training regimens, knowing the ideas must be modified moment by moment, depending upon the responses of the client.

It's like a center fielder running down a deep fly ball with two men on base. He's got to focus on the task at hand, con-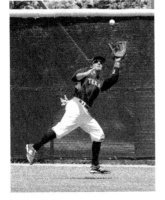tinually adjust his speed and direction, spot the ball, and know exactly when to extend his glove to attempt the catch. All the while, the batter is running and the base runners are tagging up, preparing to possibly advance bases after the catch. The fielder's teammates are moving strategically in order to guide the next move. They will align and relay the throw to the right base.

What the student-interns learn from the clients may be true education. As Robinson described high-performing educational systems ("How to Escape Education's Death Valley" 2013), they are engaged as individuals and as a team as they are encouraged to express their curiosity, individuality, and creativity in the daily client-trainer interactions. From Einstein's perspective, "What a person thinks on his own without being stimulated by the thoughts and experiences of other people is even in the best case rather paltry and monotonous" (*Jungkaufmann* 1952). The following stories obtained from the student-interns confirm the perceived effectiveness of this extended learning environment. Listen to their stories and hear sounds of genuine character development in these future leaders.

Sarah F. submitted some good observations about her role as a kinesiology graduate and a laboratory supervisor. As an accomplished national-caliber collegiate golfer, and three-time member of the dean's list, and the fall 2015 Outstanding Kinesiology Graduate, Sarah valued her time in the LWMB:

> Helping people who have disabilities improve their health and fitness, I gained new perspective. Working with people who were unable to walk made me realize how fortunate I was. It was the first time in a long time that I had felt lucky to play golf. (Fulfer 2015)

Sarah finished her graduate studies in May 2015, fulfill-ing another set of goals including a second internship as assistant golf coach at the university as well as becoming the event

coordinator at Legends Country Club.

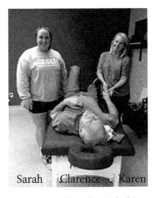

Sarah   Clarence   Karen

Sergeant Sarah with her visiting mom Karen, a registered message therapist, working with Clarence and his paralyzed right hand.

One past semester, as a collegiate track and field athlete, Sarah R. began her internship in the university weight room where she and other collegians trained for better competitive NCAA performance. Using her experience in that environment, her responsibilities, along with other interns, included developing and supervising perfor-

mance training programs for all NCAA sports.

After a week, Sarah came to the LWMB and inquired about the prospect of using training concepts on disabled individuals similar to the training for NCAA athletes but at a lower intensity. I needed nothing more than the look on her face, raised eyebrow, and wrinkled forehead to approve her request. She joined the LWMB student-intern team and became another unique talent working with disabled clients. Some clients and peers referred to her, lovingly as Sergeant

Sarah as she provided her own sort of motivation and encouragement. Her unique model taught us all another lesson, that genuine care and concern for clients permits different training styles.

Chris and Shelana served as graduate assistant leaders in the LWMB for the past year. Chris had a passion for playing football; he remembered his mom getting him up after going to sleep in his football uniform. As a walk-on, he earned a scholarship to play NCAA football

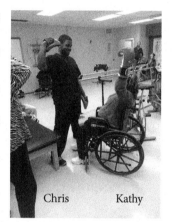

Chris   Kathy

Boxing exercise with
Chris and Kathy

player at 375 pounds. As a center on the offensive line, Chris had leadership responsibilities as well as a duty to block similar-sized elite athletes, which he did with an obvious degree of ferocity. After graduating, Chris trimmed to 275 pounds, scaled back his intensity, and now is a kind soul supervising training in the LWMB. His intensity and his selflessness are apparent as he is focused on helping our clients regain health and fitness.

Shelana, a motivated model of health and fitness was known for her encouraging push for improvement. From their very diverse backgrounds, they provided not only genuine examples of personal wellness and dedication to training, but they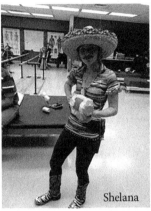

Shelana
Fun on Halloween

also exemplified the Einsteinian ideal of "pleasure in work, pleasure in its result, and the knowledge of the value of the result to the community." This model of leadership resonates through the LWMB.

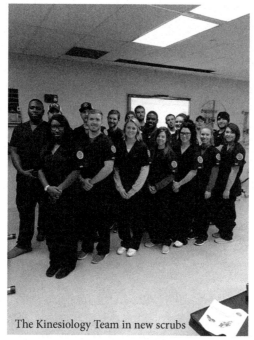

The Kinesiology Team in new scrubs

First Semester in the new LWMB KINE174
with the spring 2015 trainers

During the spring 2015 semester, thirteen undergraduate students volunteered to serve three hundred hours each
in the LWMB. The group was comprised of seven women and
six men with an average GPA of 3.38 ± 0.21 with a range of 2.5
to 3.59 on a 4.0 scale. The young pre-professionals expressed
interest in careers in rehabilitation, including occupational
and physical therapy, physician assistants, and in biomedical laboratories. They collectively administered training

programs to forty-eight individuals who otherwise would be overlooked or unserved by the conventional health-care system. The student-interns as client Irene observed, "come from different backgrounds and they have different plans."

Subjective evaluations of their value to the LWMB suggest that rather than being GPA-related, they contribute to the health of clients through their positive and genuine support of their recovery. Numerous responses to training experiences in the lab reveal some of this support.

Student-intern Bailee played collegiate softball in the NAIA and the NCAA but only after long periods of preparation and dedication. She said, "I really had to focus on what I wanted and how I was going to get there. After a year of small-college softball, I walked on to the NCAA field and became the starting catcher." Following an outstanding experience in collegiate sports, Bailee described her role in the LWMB:

It's incredible to be able to be a part of some of the life changing steps we are seeing. Words can't even begin to describe how proud I am of the clients this week. Each week that I get an opportunity to work with our clients, I see them getting strong mentally and physically. I am surrounded with an awesome staff and incredible clients. I am truly blessed with such an amazing opportunity. (Mauldin, Google+ 2015)

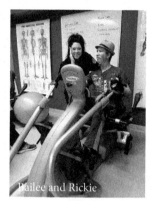

Bailee and Rickie

A special bond develops between trainers and clients.

Five weeks into the training program Bailee added:

Working with our clients isn't just about the physical gains they are making, but the mental strides as well. Working with our clients begins to show you just how amazing and interesting each of them truly are. Each client has a story to tell about themselves and the journey they are on. We are seeing such amazing progress from our clients. We have started to really challenge them individually in the lab by changing up their workout routines and cranking up the resistance and reps. Each of our clients has goals that are so specific and unique to them that it is truly special to help them accomplish this. By continuing to get our clients out of their comfort zones and working together, we help them reach new goals. (Mauldin, Google+ 2015)

Student-intern Doyle told of his interaction with Monte, modifying training routines according to the challenges that Monte faces every day.

He has been having several issues with his shoulder lately. I have been working with him a lot on the web slide exercise rail, he has his normal routine but I have been altering his routine to change things up and keep him moving forward in the right direction, as well as increase strength and mobility in his gleno-humeral joint. He says he is already noticing a difference in how his shoulder is feeling during his day-to-day activities. We're making great progress. (Dawes 2015)

Student-intern Colton and future coach recognized:

My internship in the Wellness Lab has presented many opportunities to learn new things that will further my career. In the lab I've learned that each person is unique and has their own story. Learning that means that I have to deal with them differently. In coaching there will be times a coach has to deal with emotions and skills of individual athletes in order to get them motivated and determined.

Also in the wellness lab I've learned that working together in most situations is better than working alone. In addition to what I've already learned I would also like to learn easier and more efficient ways to better the clients. Dr. Priest has given us great ideas on equipment and tools we can design in order to better our clients. This week in the lab taught me the importance of surrounding yourself with those that will stick with you through adversity. (Rheinlaender 2015)

Colton added:

Today, Dr. Priest spoke with me about the muscles that are agonists in ankle eversion and inversion while I worked on Rickie's ankle. I found it interesting how I could feel the peroneus muscles contracting even though there is a lack of control. Rickie also walked down the hallway, without his cane, in two minutes and seventeen seconds which left a smile on my face all week. Joel is making great progress with being able to get range of motion through his hips.

Colton's leadership skills expanded daily, as he interacted with multiple clients and fellow trainers.

Dustin was a student-intern looking forward to attending graduate school in the future. His experience in the LWMB proved to be valuable beyond his expectations.

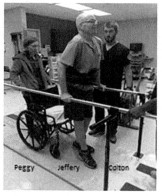

Jeffery during gait training in parallel bars with Trainer Colton and wife Peggy following with chair.

This could not be more beneficial for me right now as I am able to learn what works and try many different activities on our clients. I am also very thankful that the clients I am working with are so open to my ideas and so willing to work on different things just to see some progress. Even though I have only been in here a short time, I have already seen some amazing improvements in so many that come in. I am glad that I am able to do this internship before I go to graduate school because I feel like it will prepare me for my future both in school and in my career as an Occupational Therapist. (Blevins 2015)

Most students who volunteered for internships in the lab were kinesiology majors, but Ebun was a major in Biomedical Laboratory Science. After a few tentative days in the lab, her confidence grew. She said:

I really feel that interning in this lab was one of my better decisions, I love being able to work with others and help them improve themselves. When I'm interning, I know everything I do has a greater purpose. This week has been filled with work and a whole lot of laughter, we've maintained a perfect balance of work and play. I feel myself getting closer to the clients because we can joke about anything while making progress and achieving our goals. The exercises I had Irene do this week was to help her range of motions on her shoulders and to get more strength in her arms. She told me what her goals were and why she wanted to get them done. I have complete faith that she will be able to carry her groceries without her walker. (Ogunola 2015)

Ebun was hesitant to try to motivate clients then later realized that she herself was becoming energized.

One of the many things that makes my day at the lab are [Client] Brandi's stories, she always has me dying of laughter. Her bubbly and carefree energy is one of the things that gets me going and keeps me motivated throughout the day. (Ogunola, 2015)

As a student intern, Travis works with several clients during the course of a week. He often gravitates to Barbara, who is especially grateful for her improvement.

Over the past few weeks I've been working more with Barbara. No matter the circumstances, she always comes to the lab with a positive and cheerful attitude. We have been using the orthotics for her right hand more often and now she has gained more movement with her index and middle finger than before. She is able to slightly extend and flex both

87

fingers. This is such a great accomplishment as it motivates both Barbara and I to work harder. We're looking forward to these upcoming weeks and seeing further results. (Boody 2015)

After a week off from ice-storm closure at the university, Alysha commented about her activities with Tony.

Keeping a positive attitude is critical in these times for both interns and patients. Tony was all smiles this week; I guess he was happy to be back and working hard. On Monday he gave me a hard time about my nail polish so I told him I was going to paint his nails black on Wednesday. On Wednesday after arguing about it he let me paint one nail black. I am so grateful that we can joke around and have fun with the patients in the lab. I believe it makes the atmosphere fun and enjoyable in the lab which helps patients and interns feel comfortable. Tony also worked very hard on Wednesday with walking and did very well. Most of the time when it comes to accomplishing goals when exercising, most of the battle is mental. Whether it is trusting that your body can handle it or sticking with it and being positive until results finally show. (Kohutek 2015)

The young (mean age of student-interns during the spring 2015 semester 21.2 ± 1.2 years) pre-professionals entered the training experience needing application and interaction skills that may not have been encountered in the undergraduate kinesiology degree.

Student-intern Julia applied her experience as a high school competitive dancer and a collegiate musician. She contributed on Google+:

What I'm hoping to learn from working in the lab is seeing different opportunities I have for my future. I know that being a kinesiology major is my calling but what do I do with it? I see a future in occupational therapy, physical therapy, and exercise physiology. What I see myself doing in the future is a fun combination of those. I still don't know what I want to with my degree but I now have a better idea.

One of her clients, before working with Julia, could speak only four words.

Another client and I worked with her on saying four new words; blue, red, green, and yellow. The entire time she was in the lab, which was about two hours, she could not only say those words but point to them if we show her the colors. She has come such a long way and I can't wait to see her future progress!

In April 2015, Julia worked with Irene on specific goals.

This week Irene brought her daughter in-law in the lab so she can see what the lab was all about! She was amazed to see how far along she has come.

Seeing Irene work on a level 7 on the NuStep, walk in the parallel bars and walk around the room with a medicine ball in a Walmart plastic bag, and working with some free weights! Her daughter in-law told me that being here in the lab has been the best thing for her and I couldn't agree more. (Mathews 2015)

The LWMB served the entire Department of Kinesiology as a model for adaptive training, which our majors were required to complete. Jaycie, now a public school teacher, visited the lab in June. This is her candid and insightful commentary, providing testimony of effective learning:

What an *amazing* group of *hard workers!* They are so much fun to talk to because they make me appreciate what I have been blessed with. These warrior stories are so inspirational, and I wish more people would take notice to their amazing accomplishments. They took what someone told them they would never be able to do again, and *did it*. (That should be *Nike's* next logo "Just did it.")

I got a chance to visit with [client] Clarence for a little bit during the class when we went to the lab, and a little here and there in the hallways and while he is waiting on his ride. He is the sweetest guy ever. It is hard to believe that he could not talk, and now we are having full blown conversations. I noticed he was wearing his big buckle and asked him how he won it, and he told me the whole story! Clarence and the rest of the wonderful people in the lab did not get there on their own. Jeff and Clarence told me one morning that they were not allowed in the lab without supervision. (Hooper 2015)

Another kinesiology major visited the LWMB on a classroom assignment:

I have been in the lab multiple times while here at Tarleton. I never really understood what exactly was done in there… I just thought it was a rehab facility or a place for students to observe and learn training techniques. After spending some more time in the lab, I realized just *what* is done in there, and how amazing some transformations are! There are people in there who were told would never walk again, and now they take the "lap" around the kinesiology offices/classrooms! People in there were told they would probably never speak again, and now they can *tell* you all about their day. A stroke victim who had no more use of their arm, now is able to do thousands of revolutions *with* their arm! It's really amazing. Had I known before what I know now, I would have made it more of a priority to work in there in some way, just to gain the experience *and* knowledge. Understanding just how the body works and just how the muscles work can help these people get their lives back… the interns and professors work together to figure out just what they need to do to get a person functioning again, or at least better than when they came into the lab! More places need facilities like this. (Hite 2015)

The LWMB supervisors for the spring semester 2015 changed. Graduation periodically took our most experienced trainers and turned them loose for their careers. As I explain this to our disappointed clients, "I can't afford them anymore." I have the opportunity to identify the next generation leaders as the student-interns complete their three-hundred-hour training activities, and from that group, I am able to select the next leaders. After graduation, they become eligible to become graduate assistant supervisors in the LWMB. The monetary reward in less than ten thousand dollars per year, but it keeps them in the university environment where they have faculty mentors with various areas of expertise.

I asked client Irene, from whom I often get inspiration, on one occasion how I was ever going to replace these outgoing interns. Her immediate insightful response explains my admiration for her, "Oh, they'll find you."

Sure enough, Courtney found us and volunteered for the summer internship in the LWMB. Focused on entering physical therapy school after graduation, she gravitated quickly to a key position of leadership, providing obvious positive influence on clients and peers. After three weeks, she commented, "I have gained incredible knowledge and experience already from my time interning in the Laboratory of Wellness and Motor Behavior. More than anything, I have found a new respect for people with disabilities" (Spitzer, Student/Intern 2015).

Summer 2015 student-interns applied their ever-increasing understanding of human movement potentials in training activities in the LWMB while they pursued their other curricular requirements.

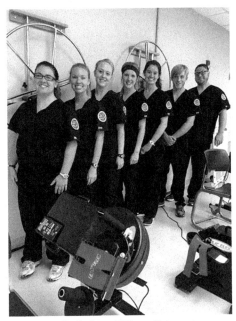

Sarah, Shelana, Hillary, Courtney,
Lauren, Haden, and Austin

These student-interns continued uninterrupted training activities for fifteen returnees and five new clients. Each trainer specifically chose to complete 225 hours, making special individuals achieve better wellness and motor behavior. Who wouldn't be happy working under the direction of these overachievers?

Courtney chose the LWMB internship because she recognized:

the opportunity was unlike anywhere else, and it turned out to be more than I ever thought it would be. It has made me aware that the same exercise on two different people will have different outcomes... and sending patients home after six weeks of therapy is not the solution. (Spitzer, Student-Intern 2015)

She quickly adjusted to helping clients in the lab; her quiet, deliberate approach created a relaxed and pleasing interaction among trainers and clients. In her typical intuitive style, she reported:

Last week I found a new respect for people with disabilities; more specifically stroke survivors. After we finished his workout for the day, Clarence sat on the stretching table to rest until it was time for him to meet his wife outside for lunch. While sitting there, he was staring at his right hand in the orthotic. I noticed him pulling his thumb away from the rest of his fingers and then thinking hard to force it back toward them again. I watched him do it for a few minutes and then he looked up at me with a big smile and said "it's getting stronger." I've watched the clients for weeks now struggle to do some of the smallest things, but until I heard the pride in Clarence's voice for seeing improvement in something as small as adducting his thumb, I didn't truly appreciate how hard clients like Clarence work in the LWMB for even the smallest progress. This work is amazing! (Spitzer, Google+ 2015)

Courtney recognized very early that will stay at the university after her internship to finish courses required for her entry into professional school. Asked about a suitable replacement for her next semester, she said, "They need to be dedicated to making people better and nothing else." Courtney has made us better.

The attitude was infectious. Each semester, even with a new group of interns, the lab gravitated to a very positive and enjoyable environment. People collectively helping people seemed to bring out the best in everybody. Lauren said:

I love coming up with exercises that will benefit each client in their own special way. I introduced Clarence to squats so that he can get in and out (mainly out) of his recliner easier. The clients love it when they know that the exercises that we are pre-scribing have a personalized purpose. (Finley 2015)

Finishing the summer 2015 semester, Sara B. contributed:

This whole semester in the lab I learned how big of an impact my fellow interns have been on my suc-cess. We have been able to work side by side with each other to get the best out of our clients and we each bring new ideas for them... I have learned the importance wherever my career takes me to contin-uously learn from others around me in the work-place. (Bollinger 2015)

The growth tendencies for the LWMB continued into the fall 2015 semester when thirteen students chose to complete their degree requirements by volunteering three hundred hours of service to forty-three individuals who needed special adaptive physical training.

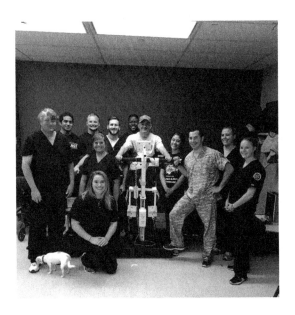

Pictured above with client Blaine (and Scooter), the new student-interns are ready to accept the challenge of improving the wellness and motor behavior of the new and returning clients. Showing off their black scrubs, Blake sports his camo scrubs, representing the university's Reserve Officers' Training Corps (ROTC) program.

After the first few days of training, the general managers began to contribute to our Google+ site. Their feedback provided us with insight into the benefits of the Applied Learning Experience. Bailee, who chose to volunteer another three hundred hours to the LWMB as a new graduate student said, "It is week one here in the LWMB and words cannot describe how truly impressed and excited I am to see the amount of progress just from my last semester to work in the lab" (Mauldin, Google+ 2015). After only a week in her new intern assignment, Emily noted:

> I can't even begin to explain how great of a decision this internship was for me... I have seen so many patients open up and get so excited about coming into the lab that it makes me excited to be there every day. (Stock, Google+ 2015)

More evidence of the value Student-interns place on the experience in the LWMB came from Chandler:

I met Gabe for the first time this week and got to work with him. I didn't get a chance to learn his story until Chris walked in the room. The excitement that Gabe had when he saw Chris was unbelievable. Gabe kept telling me, "that's Chris, that's Chris!" Chris came and sat down, and Gabe started letting tears roll down his face. He was so happy to see Chris again. It was an amazing experience to witness, and I will never forget it. The lab never ceases to amaze me. (Snodgrass 2015)

Student-intern Jamie, demonstrates her dedication to and appreciation of the LWMB. While she also takes care of her husband, raises three of her own children, and completes her final semester of curricular responsibilities, she manages to care for clients and celebrate their successes. "This makes me so happy to see all the improvements, and to see the happiness on our clients faces when they do something they haven't done in so long" (Clark 2015). Elizabeth celebrated with Jeffery, who came to us unable to stand "when he broke another walking record—walking the kinesiology base path in 6:46! He just keeps on improving every day. On the weekend he walked .88 miles at the Park and then on Sunday he walked 1.34 miles with his walker" (Cisneros, Google+ 2015).

The entire staff shared more good news as Jeffery reported walking 0.4 miles in the park using two canes instead of his walker (Moore 2015). The relationships grew between trainers and clients; they spent hours together working toward individual goals. Student-intern Victoria came from a Fort Worth Catholic High School, played club volleyball, attended a year of nursing school, visited the LWMB, and then decided that's what she really wanted to do. Soon after she started her Internship with us, client Irene told her that she loved coming here because she works out with her best friends. That was a pivotal moment for Victoria. She commented on another instance outside the university:

On Wednesday during lunch break I went up to Subway. [client] Bill had just sat down to eat. I sat with him and ate lunch with him. It was nice to get to know him outside of the lab. We got out of the environment of trainer and clients. He showed me how to open chips with one hand. I sometimes forget how much a stroke can alter someone's life. (Mamach, Google+ 2015)

I want to be able to work in a lab like this as a career, where I can work with a person for years, if necessary, to help improve their quality of life. I will go anywhere to have a career in a LWMB. (Mamach, Student-Intern 2015)

Student-intern Blake represented a different student population. He has been active in the university ROTC program. He was commissioned as a second lieutenant in the United States Army after graduating in December 2015. He planned to serve four or more years and then continue his education. His leadership skills became apparent as he began to work with clients in the LWMB. He observed:

Early in the semester, expanding our university resources, we initiated contact with Ms. McKeehan, a Registered and Licensed Dietitian, whose classes are in the Kinesiology Building. Jeffery and Randy have both had conversations with her... good to have this resource on our side. With her knowledge, this helps us and the clients get... a healthier eating habit... a nice workout routine. A healthy diet means a stronger and healthier client. The lab and clients just continue to amaze me with the life changing things that are going on within the LWMB. (Bill, Google+ 2015)

October 12, 2015 was a red letter day in the LWMB when officials from the Texas A&M University System came to visit the lab. Chancellor John Sharp and Regent Robert Albritton spent part of the morning talking with the staff and listening to the clients. Student-interns reported their impressions: Jaimie said, "It was the best feeling being able to see the pride on the clients' faces when the Chancellor asked them questions about their progress in the lab" (Hernandez 2015). Emily added, "I think the patients were definitely more excited about the whole thing than anyone else (except for Dr. Priest of course)" (Stock, Google+ 2015). Blake said, "I hope we leave a positive impact because this will open the door for everyone that's in the LWMB" (Bill, Google+ 2015).

In her second semester of voluntary service to the LWMB, the former outstanding collegiate student-athlete Bailee "learned a lot about the mental portion to our program. It is amazing what it can do for our clients and their workouts… we are changing the game up so they can become independent again" (Mauldin, Google+ 2015). A reflection of the positive attitude that prevails in the LWMB came from Chris: "We just got a new client who I'm looking forward to seeing his progress. He's coming to us in a wheelchair but we will get him walking soon enough!" (Edge 2015).

My point in the rather personal treatment of the student-interns was to identify and characterize them, to highlight their capabilities, their expectations, and ongoing perceptions of the three-hundred-hour educational experience. Our team approach to rehabilitation continued to gain momentum, and the success stories with evidence grew. The review of the successive groups of outstanding general managers stopped at the time of this writing.

The individuals who represented the LWMB at the tipping point did not get the recognition they deserved. When it came to game time, the spring 2016 student-interns were always at the top of their game—prepared, ready, and willing to show off our team effort.

Bailee Mauldin

Elizabeth Cisneros

Cameron Bowyer

Rylie Chappell

Deanna Dallal

Stacey Flores

Kaitlyn Gaston

Shon Gibson

Chelsea Graham

Tandranika Johnson

Sierra Kash

Jordan Larkin

Corey Schroeder

Kelly Isom

Seth Hallmark

Raven McGrath

Taylor Watts

Sammy Chavez

Falysha Williams

Gabriel Perry

The feedback from these volunteer student-interns can be viewed online.[2]

Without the very positive relationship between and among the staff and clients, the culminating Applied Learning Experience would not be suitable. As a professor, I had the opportunity to teach them in the classroom and then to watch

---

2   https://plus.google.com/u/0/communities/112013677417890
     656684?cfem=1.

them grow as they applied their knowledge to real people, an incredibly gratifying experience for me. What a great experience for the young men and women who are going to assume positions of leadership in our country. I just hope to hang around long enough to see the changes that will occur in the World Series of exercise training under their direction.

After Graduation?

Many of the former general managers expressed interest in a career where they could continue to provide wellness and motor behavior training for individuals who have been released from conventional care. At the time of writing this, no similar career opportunities existed for the former supervisors of the LWMB. Following graduation, they became professionally productive in many different fields, some of whom are highlighted below.

Donny Bruce completed research for his master's degree as he served as LWMB graduate assistant in 1996/7. His thesis was "Electromyographical Responses of Selected Muscles in Spinal Cord Injured During Psycle Training." His 1997 work implicated the potential of training paralyzed muscle. His chosen career was public school teaching.

Joe Ferguson completed his Bachelor's degree while serving as a supervisor in the LWMB in 1997/8. During his undergraduate studies he competed research activities that he presented at the national conference of the American College of Sports Medicine entitled "Electromyographic Responses in a C7 Tetraplegic During Passive Leg Cycling." His career choice was in the health and fitness industry.

Dee Hargrove was a graduate assistant in the LWMB in 1998/9, completing his master's degree in physical education. During his studies, he collaborated with faculty and peers that culminated with four presentations at state conferences of the Texas Association of Health, Physical Education, Recreation, and Dance. His career choice was public school coaching and teaching.

Lindsay earned her master's degree in 1999 while she was a graduate assistant in the LWMB. She was responsible for one national and two state conference presentations of her training activities. In 2008, she completed her PhD in kinesiology at the University of Houston. Dr. Edwards continued her service as a tenured associate professor in Fitness and Sport Sciences at Hardin-Simmons University in Texas.

Casey Balkenbush supervised the LWMB in 2004/5 during his graduate studies. His research activities focused on the response of spinal cord injured subjects to exercise training. He presented findings at the national conference of the ACSM in Nashville, Tennessee, entitled "Effect of Arm-Powered Passive Leg Cycling on Heart Rate Variability in Spinal Cord Injured Individual." After completing his master's degree, he continued to work toward his PhD at Texas Woman's University in Denton. He continued to have an intense interest in exercise science and is employed as a public school teacher.

Mark Hayworth, BS, MS, RN was a trainer in 2007 in the LWMB prior to beginning his master's degree. He completed a 2008-graduate credit course in Advanced EKG Studies, that spurred interest in a clinical career. His research activities included heart rate variability changes with body position and exercise. He transferred to East Stroudsburg University in Pennsylvania, where he completed his master's degree in clinical exercise physiology. Mark returned to Tarleton where he completed another degree in 2014 as a registered nurse. At the time of this writing, Mark was employed at the Level One Trauma Center at John Peter Smith Hospital in Fort Worth.

Russell Gardner completed a case study as an undergraduate working in the LWMB. He published an abstract in *Medicine and Science in Sports and Exercise* in 2002 entitled "Effects of Repetitive Movement on the Electromyographic Response of the Triceps in a C-5 Tetraplegic." These early findings provided additional basis for the use of passive training of paralyzed muscle.

Chris Hearell served as the graduate assistant in the LWMB in 2012 and 2013. After completing his master's degree in kinesiology, he planned to be accepted in Officer Training School and become a pilot in the United States Air Force.

The Players—Clients in the LWMB

The clientele encountered in the LWMB have typically exhausted their medical and therapeutic care and have approval from physicians to participate in training. The clients who took advantage of the supervisory train-ing represented students, who got

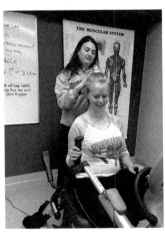

Christina and Chelsea
Never, never, never give up.

priority positions in the training schedule, members of the community and surrounding area, and recently included our first wounded warrior, a veteran of both Viet Nam and Afghanistan. He was an exciting addition because he represented some of the forty thousand veterans in the US who had limited access to recovery efforts.

The following stories came from the individuals and family members who were happy to visit while they trained and shared their fascinating histories. We took time to get to know them, and behind their disability, we found very enjoyable and even entertaining characters. Some of their stories are chronicled in order to provide the reader with insight into the particular time line in their recovery. The clients were very agreeable to the idea of retelling their stories so that others in similar situations may regain hope. They often revealed their desperation and expressed how easy it would have been to simply give up after being released from conventional care with little hope. If you listen intently to these stories, you can just make out what they're saying. One client related to me that the saddest day of his life was not when his stroke took away his family, his independence, and his job, but it was when being released from three weeks of therapy, his therapist's parting words were "There's nothing more we can do" (Pratt 2015).

The stories with evidence from this representative group of clients in the LWMB, as Dr. Rediger (A Medicine of Hope and Possibility 2015) suggested in his TED talk, "need a platform because these stories inspire people and people who are inspired overcome barriers and then inspire others. As we create pathways of health and vitality, others find and create their own pathways."

Jerry—Cerebral Palsy

On Wednesday, after two days of icing closure of the university, conspicuously, Jerry met me inside the front door, smiling from his motorized buggy, showing four fingers. I was thinking, "Is it four days of record workouts, or the Texans basketball team won by four points?" No hint from Jerry. After my obvious missed point, he explained that that day he would complete his 2,400th workout. As a testament to his endurance and the viability of the LWMB training model, client Jerry had continued his activities for more than twenty-one years. In 1994, I gave him a simple, moderate exercise prescription straight from my corporate past at the Cooper Institute for Aerobics Research—three to four days per week of continual exercise at 65–80 percent of maximum heart rate for twenty to thirty minutes per day (Cooper, Aerobics 1968). Cooper encouraged "train not strain" and assured that anyone who follows the principles outlined in his 1982 book would live a happier, healthier, and more productive life (*The Aerobics Program for Total Well-Being* 1982). In a later book, he added that indoor cycling would be another way to accomplish aerobic training without weight-bearing and joint strain (Cooper, *Running Without Fear* 1985).

Jerry had been unwavering in his dedication to training, mostly on the Psycle (IntelliGEN, Wichita Falls, Texas), an energy-regeneration, direct-drive, recumbent leg cycle ergometer. A monitor, visible to the client and the trainers, continually counted his revolutions, showed his current pedaling rate, heart rate, and power output as well as providing an estimate of his time to completion of his prescribed workout. He routinely worked above his 75-percent maximum heart rate at a perceived exertion of eight to nine (on a one to ten scale from easy to hard).

The results obtained from Jerry's training diligence over twenty-one years were remarkable. His cerebral palsy (CP) had not prevented him from being a regular as well as an inspiration to others with similar exercise restrictions. A 2009 Danish study of the lifetime health-care costs for CP for men in his age group was about 860,000 euros (over one million US dollars) (Kruse 2009). Another study in America identi-

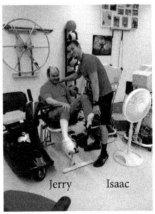

Jerry   Isaac

fied annual health care expenses for children with CP to be $15,047 higher than children without CP (Kancherla 2012).

Jerry made no big deal out of his health, but I had quizzed him for the duration of our training activities. He spent very little on health care— he was seldom sick, he had no aller-

After 2,400 cardiovascular workouts, "I will continue to train here as long as you let me," a testament to Jerry's loyalty and humility.

gies, no sore throats, no sore back, or orthopedic problems. I had never heard him cough or seen him discouraged; he was always pleasant and after all those years, knew most of the answers to my kinesiology questions that I fired at the trainers. Student-Intern Ty noted:

> Jerry is dedicated to make-up for his missed workouts [due to ice and university closure—my words]. At the end of this week he will accomplish over 2,400 workouts. That's absolutely amazing and I think we can all learn from him about his dedication to the lab. (Caruso 2015)

In the spring of 2016, Jerry completed his 2500 workout goal. He was excited about that because the university president agreed to come to the lab and watch that occasion. Semester after semester, Jerry continues to amaze, he is an inspiration.

Mike—Quadriplegia

Another client, Mike, has trained in the LWMB on and off for fifteen years. As a Texas bull rider, he competed for eighteen years in numerous rodeos. According to Mike, after leaving a mad bull, he fractured the fifth and sixth vertebrae in his neck (C5 and C6) at a rodeo in the West Texas Town of El Paso. Surgery stabilized his cervical spine and fused the C5 and C6 vertebrae; more fusion down to T1 followed years later. As a quadriplegic, he lost feeling below the injury and control of most of his skeletal muscles. That paralysis left him with voluntary control of his head, still able to move in all directions, limited shoulder movement; he could not extend his elbows or move his forearm or hand against gravity.

Conventional training generally centers on strengthening and using the upper extremities (Sherrill 1993). Following 2.5 months of conventional rehab therapy, he was released from health care and returned home. In personal discussions, Mike described his wife leaving and the depression and drug use that followed. He fell through the cracks of the American health-care system and by his admission, floundered for years.

In 1999, he learned of our LWMB program from John, a wounded Dallas policeman and former LWMB client. Mike trained with us for about two years, learning how to accomplish independent exercise on the Psycle (IntelliGEN, Wichita Falls, Texas). This helped him:

A lot mentally, and putting out the effort and getting results restored his confidence and hope… but I lost control, got another divorce, went wild, and again turned to drugs. This was followed by a bunch of negatives, including pressure sores, blood pressure and dehydration issues, and bad diet. Family does not want to be around you. Prescription pills are easy to get and have a lot of effect on your life. Methamphetamines were my choice again. (Godfrey 2015)

He tried other wheelchair sports after his injury but was not athletic at 230 pounds and seemed to fail at everything. Michael Phelps had just won eight Olympic gold medals, and that motivated him again. He began training again with the LWMB trainers, that time leg cycling then swimming. Student-intern Bryan, a university cross-country athlete, became his trainer two to five days per week. Bryan added the spark that started Mike's rally. With very few active muscle groups, Mike eventually swam thirty-two laps (sixty-four lengths) of our Olympic-sized pool, losing seventy pounds in the training process.

The Paralympic Games in North Dakota gave Mike a noble target in the 200–m backstroke, which he won, hoping to qualify for the World 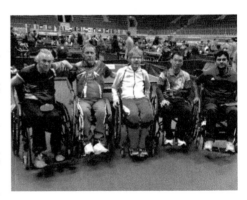 Paralympic Games in London, United Kingdom. Even with the disappointment of not making that trip, Mike was very athletic at his new post-competitive swimming body weight of 178 pounds, and he became very energized. Competing in a different sport, he qualified in table tennis for the Parapan American Games in Toronto. That international competition suited him fine, and he is now motivated to continue training. What a comeback. Mike is another great inspiration and role model for individuals who have severe limitations in movement.

Blaine—Quadriplegia

A welder by trade, Blaine rode bulls for fifteen years. He decided to return to college at thirty-one years old. He was an able-bodied student for two years and completed his sophomore requirements. On July 9, 1995, when competing at a local rodeo, a bull kicked him in the back of the neck and bruised his spinal cord at the C5–C6 level.

I remember everything—never lost consciousness. As soon as I landed on the ground, I moved my left leg for about two seconds before it went limp. I knew what had happened; I felt nothing below my neck, but I was in great pain at the point of the injury. The paramedics did an excellent job getting me out of the Stephenville arena and getting me via Care Flight to Harris Methodist Hospital in Ft. Worth. In three weeks of acute care, they took bone from my left hip to fuse C5-C6, I contracted pneumonia, had two bronchoscopies, and I was made comfortable with heavy doses of morphine. After three weeks of sub-acute care, Care Flight delivered me to a Houston rehab center. (Manigold 2015)

This consummate rodeo cowboy had many frustrations during rehabilitation, mostly because he still wanted to be treated like a bull rider. "They mostly trained me on how to be a quadriplegic," he said. Having been a student in exercise physiology and understanding critical drug side effects, Blaine took himself off all medications during the fifty-four days at the institute, with the exception of Ditropan (oxybutynin), a medication taken to reduce muscle spasms of the bladder. He often subjected himself to additional workouts "after hours because I didn't think the training was as intense as it should be."

Most SCI individuals with similar C6–C7 injuries have annual medical care expense of about fifty-four thousand dollars (University of Alabama 2006). Over one two-year period, Blaine said, "I spent six dollars for an antibiotic for a bladder infection. After 20 years, I have probably saved the American Health Care System ¾ million dollars." He, like most other SCI patients, took Baclofen (Lioresol) to reduce muscle spasms. The thought at the time was that spasms could be dangerous to him and helpers during transfer and other movement efforts, increasing the risk of falling or being dropped. "I talked to the doctor about weaning myself off the drug, and he said that it would be all right as long it did not endanger myself or others. At this point, I'm taking no medications," he said with a note of personal pride.

At his release from sub-acute care, Blaine also spoke with pride on his independence. Six months post-injury, he returned to school in January 1996 to finish his BS degree in kinesiology and take advantage of the LWMB training opportunity.

Blaine's resilience had been remarkable throughout his training program at and about the LWMB. Volunteer student-interns transferred him from motorized wheelchair to the Psycle (IntelliGEN, Wichita Falls, Texas). His original training activities involved strapping his torso and feet to this direct-drive, energy-regenerating recumbent leg cycle ergometer. Trainers provided power for leg cycling by applying enough force to the pedals to overcome the ten-watt power requirement. For continuous cycling, that required an average force of about two pounds, which the trainers were able to provide for extended periods. His training time was gradually extended, eventually reaching three thousand revolutions per training session and alternating multiple trainers. Blaine noted that swelling in his ankles went away, and he knew that it was due to his activities on the leg cycle ergometer. He noticed improvements, not only physiological but also psychological, which turned out to be a lifesaver as his wife soon left him.

After an SCI, cardiovascular control is compromised because of impaired control of the autonomic nervous system, leading to low blood pressure (hypotension), slow heart rate (bradycardia), concerns for deep venous thrombosis, long-term risk of cardiovascular disease, and susceptibility to autonomic dysreflexia (AD) (Krassioukov 2012). Tethered to the pedals, Blaine's response heart rate to the passive exercise was typically 110–120 beats per minute with no apparent exertional stress.

After several months of training three days per week, Blaine said, "Get away and watch this." He had figured out how to power the rotary motion of the pedals without assistance. At a ten-watt power setting on the ergometer, his heart rate rose steadily with this independent exercise. I quizzed him for an explanation of how, as a C5–C6 quadriplegic, he was able to accomplishing this without help. As a graduate of the department of kinesiology, he offered an impressive impromptu answer:

My biceps are normally innervated and I have a little wrist extension, so on the recumbent cycle, I can reach my right arm under my right leg and pull enough to initiate pedal motion; then similarly on the left side, alternating for continuous motion. I pull on my leg with pulls on the ankle which pulls on the pedal which pulls on the crank arm which powers the Psycle. (Manigold 2015)

Once again, his training time was extended and his intensity was gradually increased, eventually reaching one thousand revolutions per training session, and alternating arms-pulling-on-legs. He no longer needed the torso strap to secure him on the Psycle; he had gained enough stability to feel very secure in the saddle. We frequently observed Blaine working with great effort at 160 beats per minute. Blaine said, "I feel very good working at 145 beats per minute for 30 minutes, which is a complete workout for an able-bodied man my age. I don't feel like I have muscle atrophy like many other quadriplegics have."

Others with similar disabilities may identify with Blaine, talking about his experiences brought on by his spinal cord injury. He has experienced, like most other individuals who have cervical spinal cord injuries, episodes of AD. This is a cardiovascular reaction of the autonomic nervous system causing among other things sudden onset of excessively high blood pressure, severe pounding headache, and sweating above injury level (Healthwise Staff 2014). Blaine describes one such event when he had those symptoms while at home at 10:00 p.m.: "I felt every beat of the heart; I knew what it was, I just couldn't fix it." Knowing of the danger that excessive blood pressure above lesion level could cause a stroke, he drove himself to the emergency room where, with no apparent humility, "I diagnosed my problem to the doctors" as a blockage in his urinary drain tube. That, he explained, was a result of stones that had developed in his bladder that had passed out of the bladder and became lodged at a bend in his external urinary drain tube. Blaine pointed out that the doctors were somewhat impressed that a bull rider had that kind of education. Through his years of training, the trainers successfully dealt with other AD episodes, one involving new jeans that had been cinched up too tight, and another where a new shoe had been laced too tight. Blaine had typical responses to both of those, and they were successfully corrected by the trainers with no further complications.

Always ready to help others in similar situations, he explained that he had a supra pubic catheter surgically inserted (under general anesthesia), for convenience that allowed him to live alone, "and go on vacation. I would suggest that anyone who can self-catheter might not like this permanent solution—it never completely heals and needs a little cleaning," Blaine explained.

Now, somewhere past half a million revolutions on the Psycle, he enjoys a drug-free and an unusual if not incredible level of health. He credits much of his success to other quadriplegics who trained side by side on another Psycle. The friendly competition between him and Daniel, a competitive gymnast, was constructive for both of them. A by-product of the exercise habit is weight control. At 156 pounds and high energy, less body weight on the chair and the cycle saddle, the susceptibility to pressure sores disappeared. Transfers became easier.

After nineteen years of train-ing, Blaine has gained an impressive degree of independence; he lives on his own with daily nurse visits, prepares meals, eats a reasonably healthy diet, and has driven his own van since 2003. He is proud to tell of his two-week trip to Yellowstone Park by himself, driving and staying at hotels all along the way. Somewhat

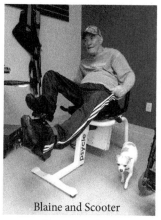

Blaine and Scooter

Blaine, with his accomplice Scooter, trains on the Psycle where he has accomplished over 0.5 million repetitions of unassisted leg cycling.

bluntly (as he appreciates) I said to Blaine, "I've got to hear about that sometime. That could not have been easy. It must be difficult to eat a hamburger." He responded, unscathed by my comment, "Oh, I manage. It's a little messy, but I can han-dle it. I can use a fork. Two and a half days to get there, stayed two weeks, and two and a half days to get back. Sometimes I forget to be humble. I forget that I set goals way back and achieved those goals. I don't realize what I have until I get around others who don't have what I have."

The remarkable cowboy will gladly take the challenge of demonstrating to others who have similar injuries how a special program of resilience and hard work can enhance your life. Thanks for sharing details of your impressive rally from catastrophic injury. Thanks for your testimony, Blaine.

Kristin—Spina Bifida

The prognosis given Kristin's parents was not good. According to Kristin, the hospital told her parents of a 10-percent chance of survival at birth, definitely blind, and would be unable to walk or talk because of spina bifida. As a youngster, she had a full-body brace, later reduced to a knee-ankle-foot orthotic (KAFO), then an ankle-foot orthotic (AFO). Throughout her school days, her mobility progressed to using AFO and crutches. At age eighteen, Kristin decided not to walk anymore because of the lower-back and shoulder pain.

At age twenty-two, her family moved to a college town, where she was successfully ambulating on crutches. She completed her associates of arts degree and became certified in Early Childhood Education. She tried more physical therapy at age twenty-five that included an hour "if I was lucky," of mat work for six weeks. Insurance cut her off and further therapy at a personal $180 per hour was not possible. For the next several years, Kristin was in a wheelchair. She said, "All of my friends who had spina bifida had no alternatives to improve their health, so they lost hope. They experienced the degenerative changes associated with lack of activity and they died."

Kristin's guidance from physicians was that if it hurt, you take a pill, including Tramadol, an opioid pain medication. She had taken more than the prescribed dosage, causing side effects of seizures, increased risk of suicide, and drug addiction. "I didn't consider myself depressed. I took medicine to make me sleep and if I didn't wake up, so what?" The drugs complicated an already difficult situation. Her latest issue was pressure sores, which prompted her to say to one of her fellow teachers, "I'm just going to stay home and get well." A former LWMB student intern, Kutter suggested that she try the LWMB. "I thought this university was just cows and teachers," she told him unashamedly.

At the first visit with her parents to the LWMB, she said to me, "I had my walls up although you seemed to be excited. Something about you was different, like revolutionary, very inspiring and convincing. I remember rolling into the LWMB for the first time, and my life has not been the same since."

Kristin commuted for the first three months to our lab, over ninety miles round trip, three days per week. Kristin's work ethic in the lab was incredible. Her summer and fall 2014 semesters, she accomplished 130,100 arm and leg steps, averaging over 4,000 steps per session on the NuStep. That represented a machine-calculated equivalent of about seventy-one miles. By October 2014, she walked a mile with Dr. Lancaster (a fellow kinesiology professor) and three LWMB Student-interns; an outstanding accomplishment for Kristin in any light, but especially because she had not walked with crutches for many years. As she stood in our stabilizing device (IntelliGEN, Wichita Falls, Texas), I asked what training she did to allow her to walk a mile. She immediately responded, "This standing frame, my grandfather built one for me when I was three years old. He told me my legs were weak but they were going to get stronger. The first time I stood in this frame [the OrthoSys at the LWMB], I heard his voice again saying the same thing again. I am very confident, very secure because I am surrounded by LWMB trainers. While standing, we stretch the trunk and lower back, we play catch with the medicine balls, and other mobility exercises that give me the confidence to push my limits."

I asked Kristin what she would tell others who, like her earlier friends, have no hope. She said that she would tell them about training in the LWMB. "You may not stand the first day, but you will move, and if you don't move, you lose."

By January 2015, Kristin had established herself as a consummate teacher. She brought learning aids for client Kathy, a stroke survivor who you will meet later. Kathy had no speech after her stroke, and Kristin wanted to help. She often spent two hours with Kathy identifying and speaking names of colors. Kristin had more complex flash cards she pulled out for

Clarence. He identified red hexagon, orange pentagon, green oval when prompted with colors and shapes on the card. He struggled but got most right. Kristin was thrilled to teach, and she reduced her regular teaching assignment to two days, allowing her to spend three days per week with clients in the LWMB. She is such a talented and unique educator and motivator—maybe we can find funding to add her as an adaptive assistant. She said emphatically "I love being here."

Student-interns enjoy working with Kristin—she's loud and proud about everybody's accomplishments, including her own. At her annual appointment with her neurologist in June 2015, she chose to walk into the doctor's office, which she had never done before. She said the doctor's eyes got as big as saucers, and she said "What happened to you?" Responding to the doctor's inquiry about her medications, Kristin said, "I don't take any since I started training at the LWMB." The doctor said, "Well, you don't need me anymore."

After her incredible rally and no longer under regular medical care, Kristin said, "I want this story to be motivating to others who have spina bifida. The exercise that I do in the lab is beautifully painful. My body is starting to recognize the different kinds of pain. I have to tolerate some pain knowing that the pain of exercise is temporary and the result is worth it.

Duncan—Cerebral Palsy

Remember Jerry, the record-holder for endurance at the LWMB? He now has a new challenger named Duncan. At fourteen years of age in a loving family, he has tried lots of things which had been helpful. He attended public school through the fourth grade, demonstrating very good scholastic skills. For the past six years, Duncan has been home-schooled and has missed some opportunities to train for health, lacking the trainers and equipment that public schools were able to provide. Mom Misty says, "He has been interested in training for many years." Duncan started train-ing in the LWMB in January 2015 and immediately liked the people and activities. As I interviewed his dad, Casey, Duncan was surrounded by three trainers who were playing catch with him using a small medicine ball. Intern Bailee got a trash can and held it in front of him for him to shoot baskets. He loved the activity; on Monday, we closed for Martin Luther King Day, and Duncan and his family went to Academy Sports to buy workout clothes, exactly what he wanted, using his money.

In February 2015, Duncan walked with his ankle-foot orthotics on the Gait Trainer Treadmill (Biodex Unweighing System, Vonco Medical, Rehab, and Fitness, Carrollton, Texas). Although labor intensive to prepare for training, Duncan was secured in a body harness and attached to an overhead bar, applying lift to his torso, effectively reducing the body weight. He took his first steps on the treadmill with Misty, friends, and trainers all around. We could only imagine how the first steps might have helped Duncan, but his wide smile said it all.

Casey suggested that he sees so much so much social/psychological benefit, "This is a win-win for Duncan and the trainers, who are learning real-life lessons. Many people do not know how to interact. They don't understand his behavior nor his slurred speech. The LWMB trainers are not afraid of him and treat him with kindness.

Casey added, "He likes goals, and I like the way you track activities to keep goals progressive" (C. Cumby 2015). On February 11, 2015, Duncan set a new record on the NuStep (NuStep, Inc., Ann Arbor, Michigan). He worked thirty-eight minutes on a level three for 2.75 miles, ending up at a vigorous 120 watts and 130 to 140 steps per minute. As of October 2015, he has accumulated 103,000 arm and leg steps over 56 miles. He was so eager and proud to keep improving. Misty said, "Without this program, he would have taken few steps. He is happier and has improved his outlook. The trainers are very helpful and considerate of Duncan, not limiting his training to what previous trainers have suggested that he should and should not do. He is becoming more flexible" (M. Cumby 2015).

As Duncan became more active, student-interns stood him in the OrthoSys to support him below the waist in a standing position. He enjoyed playing catch with the basketball with student interns, Ty on one ankle and Quinn on the other. Shelana and Alyssa tossed the small basketball from both sides. His next fun activity was to spike the volleyball, which went expectedly in undetermined directions with funny impact on the trainers. Misty said, "I love the way these trainers are always thinking of something else to do, in spite of being unconventional. I thinks it's awesome. I think it's really wonderful that four trainers right now are huddled around two clients, listening while one client (Kristin) is teaching another client (Kathy)" (M. Cumby 2015).

Bill—Stroke

At 8:00 a.m. on August 26, 2010, Bill had a stroke. He was a smoker for years, and that morning his cigarette fell out of his mouth; he tried to put it back in and it would not stay. He called 911 and the ambulance team gave him the Golden Hour tPA, supposedly to minimize stroke effects. Twenty-two minutes (and according to Bill, twenty-two thousand dollars) later in the Care Flight helicopter, he was at the Intensive Care

Unit a nearby Fort Worth hospital. In surgery, Bill did not know what they did, but ten days later, he was released from the hospital. They asked him to what care center he wanted to go, to which he replied, "The one that has the best rehab." He went there for a brief period where he worked under an occupational therapist (OT) and a speech therapist (ST) in a very nice room. He was there three months. One day he asked them what he just did; they responded, "You lifted your leg ten times."

"That's what I've been doing." Then he told them, "Get me out of here." They sent him home in a loaned wheelchair and told him, "You will never be able to walk again." Bill had home health available for a while, which he characterized as therapists working after hours to make more money. He called it a rip-off and fired them.

In January 2014, Bill said he was "brought to the LWMB in a wheelchair that I borrowed from the church." He arrived in that wheelchair being pushed by a kinesiology volunteer where we met him and asked him what he wanted to do. He said, "I want to walk and use my arm." We worked around his schedule for a year as he commuted to Fort Worth, taking his wife to the oncologist. A great personality and storyteller, he told of eating at Uncle Julio's where his wheel fell off his chair and several nice people took care of him. He said, "That's the day I went to Sam's Wholesale and bought my wheelchair."

After his release from conventional care four months after his stroke, student-interns began rhythmic, passive arm and leg training on the motorized Thera-Vital (Medizintechnik GmbH, Hochdorf, Germany). The machine provided initial power to move legs and arms independently, which is termed passive exercise because Bill was not providing the power to the pedals. Again encouraged by earlier findings of the value of passive exercise (D. S. Willoughby 2002), he continued to train on the Thera-Vital for another year.

Semester by semester, the new student-interns continued and modified the training routines established by the previous group of trainers. During the fall 2014 semester, Bill said "These are the best trainers we've ever had. I made relationships with most of them." He cultivated those relationships by talking to them at length about his condition, his health, and his business success as well as the friends who also trained in the LWMB. He identified with the students because he had attended and graduated from this university, being active as a spirit leader. Decades later, he continues to be a spirit leader in our lab and in the community. He calls the trainers by name and says that he tells them each good-bye at the end of each semester in person and on Facebook. The cumulative training effect was that he learned to walk behind the chair in the LWMB, and now he tries to walk around the house independently but still too shaky to try it without help.

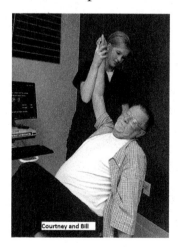

Courtney and Bill

Since those beginning efforts to accomplish continuous move-ment, Bill has adopted every new student-intern group (he has seen six different groups to date), seen every improvement, utilized every piece of equipment, and befriended every person in his contact area. I see why he is an award-win-ning business man; his communicative skills are amazing.

The past three semesters, he has utilized the NuStep favorably, completing 24,000 steps over 13.3 miles, averaging 1,200 steps over 0.7 miles. He also trained on the Psycle which allows continuous leg work, utilizing mostly the power from his unaffected leg. In three semesters of 2015, Bill completed thirty-six thousand unassisted revolutions. In his typical storytelling fashion, he reminded me of the first day he was able to accomplish an uninterrupted one thousand revolutions. "It was the day that Mr. White[3] came in for a visit to the lab with the university president. Actually, the Psycle is what got me out of the wheelchair."

By January 2015 Bill routinely walked behind and pushed his wheelchair into the building and throughout our facility, using it just for insurance. After training with us for four semesters, Bill became active in commercial real estate sales once again. In January 2014, he was awarded the Top Commercial Real Estate Producer, selling over twelve million

---

[3]   Jerry White, PE, is the author of "Six Months to Life," and wrote about his use of "Guided Imagery" in recovering from two bouts with cancer. He visited the LWMB with the hopes of collaborating with our activities.

dollars. He had previously won the award in 2013, but at that time, he accepted the award from his wheelchair. The next time, he accepted his award by walking up to the podium. "It took me a while, but I walked up there and got my award… I turned around and all the realtors were standing and applauding… pretty neat," he said with obvious emotion.

Tony—Stroke

Tony came to the LWMB in February 2014 from Afghanistan by way of Iraq. After a stroke, he could not walk, talk, or swallow. He was totally dependent upon his aging parents in their home. Student-Intern Thomas picked Tony up at his parents' house and transported him to the LWMB three times per week. He used a wheelchair inside the house, and after three months of dedicated training, described in the following paragraphs, he learned to use a walker from the house to the truck and from the truck to the LWMB.

The fall 2014, student-interns supervised a new training regimen on the newly acquired NuStep. As a former collegiate football player, Tony had no trouble facing the challenge of another method of training. During three semesters of training with as many different groups of student interns, he completed 86,500 arm and leg steps on the NuStep, covering a machine-calculated equivalent of 47.8 miles, averaging over 1800 steps and a mile per training session.

Tony graduated to training in a harness on the Biodex Gait Trainer during the fall of 2014, with overhead lift support. Although his gait was irregular and difficult, the NuStep exercise enabled Tony to accomplish a helpful smooth and continuous motion. He walked on the treadmill while watching the monitor which indicated stride length. He focused on making his stride lengths equal. It was not smooth, but he completed the six-minute test at 2.4 mph. After four training sessions, he was able to maintain balance and stride length without the harness and overhead support. His gait on the treadmill improved so that he could maintain 3.4 mph for six minutes with no overhead support but still hanging onto the full-length support bars.

It was Wednesday morning when I got to spend an hour with the LWMB troops before I went to class. It was so gratifying to see the interaction as we all strived for wellness. As I left the lab for class, I entered the busy hallway and saw Intern Thomas standing conspicuously in Tony's walker. From that situation, I was sure that Tony was somewhere within a few feet on an independent walking assignment. "Good morning," I said to Thomas, "how is Tony doing?" A young man of few words, Thomas said, "He's doing better all the time" (T. Ferguson 2015).

After nine months and three groups of student-interns doing the pickup and delivery to the LWMB for adaptive training, Tony was able to ambulate on his own. Tony's feeding tube came out in December 2014 after four years; those changes all represented significant improve-

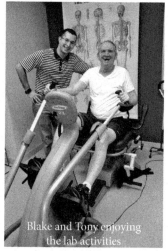

Blake and Tony enjoying the lab activities

Over 86,500 steps on the NuStep prepared Tony for improved mobility.

ments in his independence. Tony became the primary care-taker for his elderly and disabled parents in their home. By the end of the fall 2015 semester, he walked with a cane outside his house, inside the lab, and to and from the truck to the LWMB.

A player on the 1978 quarterfinalist NAIA football team, Tony was inducted with his teammates into the Athletic Hall of Fame at Tarleton State University. Tony thinks he has improved to the point where he can soon rejoin his family in the Philippines. What an impressive rally.

Rickie—Stroke

Client and stroke survivor Rickie is a formerly successful independent business owner for thirty-five years and mayor of a nearby thriving community. He recalls enjoying helping people, and he misses that now. His December 2012 stroke left him paralyzed on one side and unable to stand or walk on his own. His balance and memory was affected, and worse, his confidence was broken, and he became severely depressed. He lost his left-side peripheral vision.

He was put in an ankle-foot orthotic (AFO) and put in a wheelchair; he used a cane with difficulty since his stroke until training with us. His physical therapy (PT) at an unnamed but well-known rehabilitation facility (about six weeks of insurance coverage) was not productive. "I saw no gain whatsoever... I felt the same way when I went in and when I came out. My confidence was shot, never thought I'd get any better. They never had enough time to work with me," he recalled. They had a NuStep and he had maybe an hour of rehab if he was lucky. Very few personal relationships developed. He remained in a wheelchair and was given no hope for improvement. "Many, many times I wanted to just give up." Another rehabilitation facility, where insurance would continue to pay told him there was nothing they could do for him. Imagine the feeling of depression at that point. According to Rickie, he was suicidal within three months after his release from conventional care.

Rickie learned about the LWMB through a friend. "I like the atmosphere here—more like a club. Camaraderie personalizes the program and reinforces the work." After training with us for a year, he walked with a cane and no longer needed an AFO.

The TSU program gave me all the time I need, three days per week. Discussion with other stroke survivors was encouraged and very helpful with building confidence. Not until this program did my confidence come back. Training on NuStep and walking with trainers here increased my leg strength where I am able to walk. The encouragement is vital to improvement. The trainers have great attitudes. Future trainers must have a long range goal, not just living in the day. Sometimes, family members may have stimulated their interest. The more we get the word out on the program, the better… we need these new goals and new directions and new ideas.

After learning details about his traumatic experience with the stroke and the previous attempts at rehabilitation, Rickie's advice to me was special as I continued to strive for program recognition, "Don't let other people discourage you."

On January 30, 2015, Rickie accomplished a new goal—he walked utilizing only the walker to the car and from the car to the LWMB then after training, back to the car—left the wheelchair at home for the first time since his stroke. Up until that time, he had used the wheelchair almost exclusively. He attributed his improvement to the trainers pushing him a little further each time he comes in. I asked if his improvement was related to the NuStep, the Psycle, or the Excite™ TOP (Technogym USA Corp., Fairfield, New Jersey); he quickly responded that "the equipment is nice, but it's the trainers who make the difference. I'm on target to walking independently by the end of semester—I really think that I can get there." A few minutes later, Bailee was walking with Rickie to the parallel bars with no assistance other than a gait belt and a little support from behind.

Rickie thinks the Biodex Gait Trainer (GT) treadmill (Biodex Medical Systems, Inc., Shirley, New York) is an important tool, and he wants to use it more and graduate there to not holding the safety bars with his hands. We used unweighing about twenty pounds; more unweighing is not necessarily good because less weight on the legs increases of the tendency of twisting the ankle (supination) during gait training.

In March 2015, I asked, "What keeps you coming to the lab?"

Rickie said, "Because of the camaraderie, these kids motivate me. It makes me get up at 4:30 a.m. every day I get to be here. Sometimes I can't wait to be here" (Pratt 2015). A significant instance occurred on April 6 after Rickie walked with Intern Colton unsupported a few steps down the hallway.

Soon after on April 17, I walked up on three student-interns surrounding Rickie as he completed one hundred steps unassisted down the same hallway. Coincidentally, as we were all celebrating Rickie's new accomplishment, Joel, who you will meet later, rolled in the front door on the way to his workout. The amazement on Joel's face was priceless and provided more evidence of the importance of group interaction during training. You don't get this synergy working in isolation from others who are battling some of the same challenges or even from working in isolation with a professional therapist. The camaraderie grows undeniably with these coincidences. A reflection of his swelling pride and his growing confidence, this week Rickie donated a sacrificial sum of money to the LWMB to support operational expenses, unsolicited but greatly appreciated.

In July 2015, Hillary took Rickie to the pool for more walking practice. Soon joined by Student-Intern Sarah, the three walked ten lengths in the pool while both trainers encouraged Rickie to step the leg forward and not swing it to the side. The gait training occurs with little weight supported by the legs and lots of emotional support. With that bit of independence, he admitted that he had felt confident enough to buy a vehicle and relearn to drive, also confessing that he had practiced driving on back streets in his small home town.

He was proud to add, "I even gave my aunt a ride to the grocery store." I declare that he is over yet another hurdle.

The progress we see in Rickie is not without considerable effort on his and our part. Evidence of his continued commitment comes from his training activities on the NuStep. Through a year of recorded activities, along with his other training activities, he has accumulated over 177,000 steps covering 94 miles, averaging over 2680 steps and 1.5 miles per training session. His interpretation of his improvement: "I have been able to restore left peripheral vision, improve memory, balance, confidence, attitude, dexterity of left leg, and to regain some feeling in my left leg (Pratt 2015).

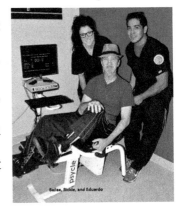

Rickie said his lab experiences contribute to his physical well-being in several ways, "Along with physical activities, there is also a need for occupational therapy, such as how to put on clothes with one hand or do chores with a disability. Thinking outside the box is a big plus in overcoming these type of everyday tasks which most people take for granted. Keep up the good work."

Unable to live independently, he lives with his dad for a while, transferring back and forth from a full-service nursing facility. *After everybody else gave up*, Mayor Rickie continues to strive for recovery after 18 months and six semesters of different student-trainer groups. His goal continues to be to be independently mobile again, and drive and work again.

Randy—Multiple Sclerosis/Stroke

In January 2012, Randy found it more and more difficult to move. Medical diagnostics could not identify a problem. The suspicion was a brain infection, and they decided to treat him with intravenous (IV) antibiotics, which was prolonged for eight months. Later, two brain surgeries revealed nothing; the third time, surgeons cut an artery causing a stroke affecting his left side. After a year, they decided on a diagnosis of multiple sclerosis (MS).

After acute care and still in a wheelchair, he went into a rehabilitation hospital for a month. He was very weak after lying around. They treated him with physical therapy one to two hours, occupational therapy (OT) one to two hours, and speech one hour per day where he showed some improvement. Walking only with great difficulty and unable to talk, he learned how to say some words. He wore a sling but took it off sometimes in therapy, but the joint never tightened or improved flexibility. Insurance dropped him after eight months. He was able to walk out of clinic in December 2013 with the aid of a cane. He wore a sling for another eight months to keep the weight of his arm from pulling his shoulder out of the socket. "I did not have the muscles to hold it in the joint," he said.

Randy started training with us in the LWMB almost immediately after his release from conventional care. At that time, his shoulder and elbow were frozen and his hand was practically useless. Immediately, the student-interns started training him on the wall wheel to get his range of motion back and then strategic strength training for the muscles that hold the shoulder joint together. Within a few training sessions, adding hand weights and bands, his shoulder was again mobile and was not dislocating. He was out of the sling permanently. Once again *after everybody else gave up*, Randy regained function and returned to work in his family business.

That did not happen with the conventional therapy but only after over a year of continuous training in the LWMB. It merits a further description of his efforts during that time. Randy was accompanied to the NuStep for training three days per week. During the next several months, Randy accomplished independent sessions totaling over 310,000 steps and 171 miles. He gravitated to the Psycle with his trainers and routinely finished one thousand revolutions requiring a relatively low-intensity forty-watt power output.

I asked Randy how he kept motivated. He replied, "I get depressed, but I come in here and see people a lot worse than me and how hard they work. I feel lucky being in here. I see how hard it is for some others to improve." Randy was the motivation for others. "I saw Clarence learning how to jog after not being able to walk. Here everybody jumps in to help.

All the trainers are good to provide help at all times." Randy described his trainers, Robert, Mallory, Chris, BJ, Sarah, James, and Shelana as outstanding. "Chris takes me to the science building to walk three hundred stairs with him." Randy summarized his comeback and described the training here as "a real confidence-builder. It gets in your mind. It's more fun, easier to come to, and the price is right. I have trainers who I can relate to… we have six to seven trainers who all help. In the LWMB, it's about a lot more than core strength, and I got my limbs back" (Smith 2015).

Kathy—Stroke

Kathy had a stroke in 2013. From the hospital and acute care, she went to a nearby nursing facility. During that time, no therapy was attempted, and mostly ignored by the staff, she sat for hours each day in the chair or on the bed. They just medicated her with pain killers, anti-depressants, blood pressure, and thyroid drugs each day. They even brought a potty-chair [sister Kay's reference to a portable commode] into the room, as she could not navigate to the bathroom. The staff of the nursing facility never encouraged her to get out of bed or to attempt standing. She did not move further than the bed to the potty-chair in the room. Having lost the ability to stand or to walk, even to talk, the idea was discussed with her two sisters that they considered hospice. Kay ended up taking her in to her home and providing care for her.

In August 2014, the sisters brought Kathy to the LWMB, where they immediately appreciated the positive and energetic environment. Sister Kay said, "Everybody is as nice, helpful, and caring as they can be." The student-interns began to work with Kathy on the wall wheel, OrthoSys (Dynamic Weight Bearing System for Spinal Cord Injured and other Disability, by IntelliGEN, Wichita Falls, Texas), along with passive arm exercise on the ExN'Flex (Model EF-100W Therapeutic Arm Exerciser, Ottawa, Ontario, Canada). Her best training sessions were over three thousand steps per day on the NuStep. In the calendar year of 2015, she completed over one hundred thousand steps and fifty-five miles. The student-interns soon gravitated her training sessions to include the parallel bars, which Kathy was able to negotiate using her hands for stability.

Kathy worked with the LWMB two days per week for 1.5 hours and one day per week in the pool, where by the end of the fall 2014 semester, she learned to walk in the water independently. During that semester, another group of trainers developed other activities, including walking with a walker in the LWMB clubhouse. By the end of that semester, she had graduated to walking with the walker on the kinesiology base path around the offices and classrooms. Kay said, "She now gets out of bed and out of her room without help, and she walks in their house using just a cane… Let's see, not long ago, we were told she was not supposed to live."

In the spring of 2015, Kathy completed six trips in

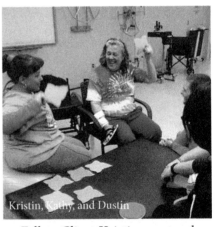

Kristin, Kathy, and Dustin

Fellow Client Kristin, a natural teacher, provides games and activities in the LWMB for Kathy to improve her motor skills and speech.

the parallel bars using no hands for the first time in three years. After the fourth trip, she literally danced at the end of the bars, smiling widely. Her prescription drug use is now reduced to her thyroid medication and an Aspirin but no more pain-relievers. "That's it, that's all she's on right now," Kay said, "and training with at the LWMB gives Kathy a purpose and a positive place to go… the training is wonderful." Many people give up after a stroke, but Kathy and her sisters tried every source and found nothing; there was no place to go—nobody would take her. Fellow client Kristin brought

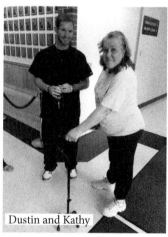

Dustin and Kathy

Walking for the first time after weeks of training in the parallel bars, Kathy walks the kinesiology base path with Student-intern Dustin.

some teaching aids from her school and started teaching new words to Kathy such as colors, numbers, greetings, etc. One day, I asked her to do something that she could not do when she first found us, "Let's hear you count," I said, to which Kathy immediately replied in a clear and distinct voice, "One, two, three…" up to ten with smiles all around. After that I asked, "How about some colors?" Kathy responded thoughtfully, with a look of determination, "One, two, three," which reminded us all of the difficulty in recovery following a stroke. She says she knows the colors but can't make the connection to say the words and often, something else comes out, much to her surprise.

By the spring semester 2015, Kathy was walking with a cane around the kinesiology base path accompanied by a student intern. She has progressed to walking independently in the house; all of this was achieved *after everybody else gave up.*

Monte- Guillain Barrè

On September 11, 2004, symptoms were instantaneous. At a fall rodeo in Salt Lake City, Utah, Monte was walking along the airport hallway when he simply fell limp. He got up the first time but fell again on the way to the hospital. He was diagnosed with Guillain-Barrè syndrome, an autoimmune disorder that attacks the peripheral nervous system and causes paralysis. In Monte's case, the paralysis was complete, even affecting his eyelids. During three months in the local hospital, he spent two hours a day in rehabilitation with the parallel bars only as the equipment.

After transferring back to Texas and admitted to a reha-bilitation clinic, he "basically laid there twenty-three hours per day... they taught me how to get along in a wheelchair. If I had not pushed myself around in a wheelchair, there was no exercise." They administered medications to him and pro-vided no hope for recovery. After a month and no sign of improvement, he was released from conventional care.

Monte began training in the LWMB in the fall semester of 2005. After little improvement from conventional care, he was excited to begin our training activities. "For my 2.5 hour training sessions, everybody is willing to work with me and help me... I've made lots of friends."

Student-interns started working on his core stability and using one-pound hand weights, which he lifted with diffi-culty. Over the next several years of continuous training (during university semesters), each successive group of student-interns worked him up from four to eight and all the way to forty-five-pound hand weights. Monte began to shoot a compound bow and even goes hunting in the Texas Hill Country. This signifies as strength of the LWMB program; the impact of the program doesn't go away. As long as Monte is motivated, we will provide necessary supervision and adaptations for training.

As a former rodeo cowboy, Monte was not afraid of hard work and when he arrived at our lab, he immediately became known for his work ethic. The calendar-2015 year,

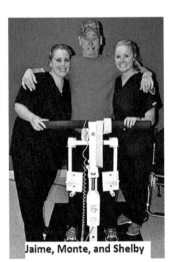

Jaime, Monte, and Shelby

The OrthoSys allowed Monte to stand while training upper-body activities

he worked diligently on the NuStep completing over 206,000 steps and 110 miles. His effort was inspiring as he averaged nearly 3,000 steps and 1.5 miles per training session. As his strength improved, he then had confidence to try standing in the parallel bars and walking in the Olympic pool, still holding onto the side for stability. Monte has gained enough stability and strength that he is now able to drive his van; an inspiring comeback from complete paralysis.

Ten years into team kinesiology training, Monte is now well and drug-free, taking only vitamins. I ask him what his goals are now: "I've got to have good trainers, and someday... I will move my legs. I've got hope now and plan on walking, roping, and hunting on my own two legs." What a resilient cowboy.

Clarence- Stroke

Clarence was a businessman in the community for thirty-five years. He had a stroke in February 2011, and he was flown to Fort Worth for critical care. As an inpatient, he worked three hours per day and three days per week for seven weeks. For the next one and a half years, he commuted (sixty miles one way) for further rehabilitation. The major stroke had taken away his ability to speak. He now remembers not being able to recognize the plumbing tools that he had been using for thirty-five years. Over that period, he progressed from a walker, he said proudly, and "walked out of therapy with a cane."

Clarence had weeks of local professional rehabilitation that he now describes as "good for a while but with no personal interaction." His wife Linda accompanied him to all training session. Upon his release, he had difficulty with balancing and walking, and he had learned to speak his numbers up to fifteen.

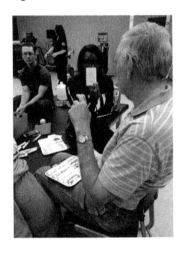 As Clarence started training in the LWMB in January 2014, his pleasant demeanor was contagious. He immediately made friends with fellow clients and trainers. I asked another client once about her motivation for continuing her training regimen in the lab. She responded, "My hero is Clarence. I want to be like him." All of that occurred in spite of his inability to speak. His response to greetings and questions was always an enthusiastic "Super," and for a while, I did

not realize his limited vocabulary. Although he was thinking clearly, he could not put the words together to communicate his thoughts.

The feeling was mutual as he described his spring 2014 trainers as "good, reliable, considerate, and understanding." His appreciation for them continued to grow, reflected in Linda's description of the trainers, "We get trainers who love to be here, and that means more than anything. It is amazing. They've got it. In regular training, you don't always get that type person. You can tell the difference from those who come because of the paycheck. I definitely see a difference. I see the camaraderie, plus all the people who train here, plus all the helpers, although they may be here for only a semester. Clarence can come in by himself, trusting that the trainers will take good care of him."

Linda said, "I get to return my life to a little bit of nor-mal. Whoever chooses these trainers must have a mold and a guideline." What she had not recognized at that time [and perhaps me either] is that the student-interns choose us. We don't choose them, and I am still not sure what constitutes a good one. Accompanying Clarence to the lab for some of the first semester." She adds, "I hope that Clarence made a difference in some of these kids, because they care about the clients. I don't know all about what he does in training, but his brain works better. I'm shocked daily that all these things are coming back. Something that is *hugh* to me is that the brain is rewiring, like they told me it would. It wasn't the same at the fitness center… there were no other stroke survivors. They were very accommodating, but that just wasn't their deal."

One gets some insight into this (tenacious?) character Clarence. After our addition of the NuStep devices, he used the stepping motion to aid his efforts at walking. Training for up to four hours each day, in seven months, he completed 207,000 steps and 110 miles, averaging 3,500 steps and almost two miles per session. For just a typical warm-up, Clarence likes to train on the Psycle five times per week. With the fall 2015 semester interns, he routinely completed three thousand revolutions each day five days per week. Able to tolerate maximum range of motion, his stronger left side provided most of the power for continuous motion. At times, the trainers would remove the left pedal, forcing the power from the weaker right side where he was able to accomplish one thousand revolutions.

Fellow client Kristin, a consummate teacher made it her objective to help Clarence talk again. Clarence said that during his recovery, he got his thoughts back before he could express them (same thing as Kathy). He acknowledged his difficulty in speaking and said his mind is working better than his speech. He thought back to after his stroke when he could not recognize his plumbing tools that he had used for thirty-five years. Clarence speaks highly of his therapist who worked with him in rehab and says she still keeps in touch with him. He says the LWMB has continually improved his mobility and his speech. "The more you talk, the better it gets, and these trainers give me a chance to talk a lot." I asked if he recognized words on the page, did he read? He said, "I read the funerals every day to see if I'm there." He asked me how we were going to adjust to being seventy years old and followed that question with "I think we just keep working." He now communicates effectively.

In the spring 2015, after more than a year of training, his trainers began to walk about one hundred meters with Clarence unassisted to the science building, where he was challenged with four flights of stairs. With two trainers at his side and no hands on the rail, he was able to go to the fourth floor, stepping up alternately with his strong and affected side.

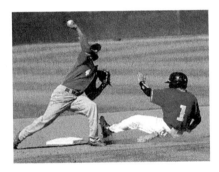

This risky idea is akin to the shortstop trying to turn the double play, knowing the oncoming base runner is sliding in, probably cleats up to break it up. The baserunner's slide threatens harm to the shortstop in order to prevent or slow the throw to first base. It is something done for the team to try to beat an opponent. The cleat mark scars on his hands and legs, suggested that Wolfe spoke with some authority (former NCAA baseball player 2015). In Clarence's case, walking four flights of stairs enabled him to overcome fear and doubt in his efforts to overcome his opponent, the lasting effects of the stroke. At the time of this writing, his goal was to run a mile, which was curious because he was not a runner prior to his stroke.

What do our overachieving interns think about Clarence? Student-intern and former athlete B. J. said it well:

Clarence is one of the most self-motivated humans I've ever met. He sets goals and achieves them with hard work. This week Clarence completed a 50-yard run and the football field and also walked the bleachers two times up and down 40 steps each. It's a blessing to be around great clients and trainers each week in the lab. (Jackson 2015)

Linda says, "I saw Clarence's concern for others growing as he trained in the LWMB. He would comment that he didn't see Bill or Brandi today, or... It's bringing back this care and

concern for *others*." The LWMB is all about people and relationships; we learn to be concerned about others like Kristin
who helped Clarence make great improvement right before
our eyes, and David, from whom Clarence used to buy hay,
and Bill, who used to deliver Clarence's propane. All of this
interaction promotes healing.

Former cowboy bull rider, client Blaine started to pay
more attention to Clarence and identified with his incredible
persistence and determination. With eighteen years of experience on the Psycle, and a BS degree in kinesiology, Blaine
respectfully requests to advise Clarence in his training activities on the Psycle. Clarence's gait progress is slow and he still
drags the weak leg. In order to stimulate his hip flexors for lift,
he advises Clarence to periodically pedal backward and pull
on the pedals instead of the more natural alternating push.
What a rewarding experience it is to see clients' concern for
each other.

Terrell and Marvin—Stroke

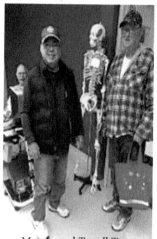

Marvin and Terrell Team

Terrell and Marvin—partners in recovery.

Stroke in these two buddies produced typical side effects. Terrell and Marvin each had one fully functioning arm and hand, which didn't make zipping up the jacket easy. Otherwise healthy, they came in three times per week to train. Their trainers supervised prescribed sessions on the NuStep where the stronger side provided power for the affected side. In nine months of 2015, they completed 265,000 and 103,000 arm and leg steps respectively. Other rhythmic movement was provided by the arm therapy device (ExN'Flex International, Ottawa, Ontario, Canada). Marvin's progress was highlighted when he reported to me that he could put a drill bit in his drill by himself, allowing him to go back to his shop. They agree that "little things become big things." He and Terrell finished workouts at the same time and with no fanfare, helped each other zip jackets prior to leaving the lab on the cool winter day. All of that was done while pleasantly smiling and joking with others in the lab.

Irene—Spinal Surgery/Paralysis

Irene's family is second-generation immigrants (grandmother) from Poland. For eighteen years, she grew up in Pennsylvania during the early 1950s to 1960s. At that time, we were in serious competition with Russia. She said, "Our teachers of English, history, math, science, etc., we definitely need to beat those guys, so lots of emphasis on achievement." She got married within three months of her high school graduation to a man in the US Air Force, where "we traveled a lot and encountered many different speaking styles. I gravitated to some more than others." Her husband uses lots of Texas slang, and Irene is sensitive to the lack of resulting communications. She learned to appreciate good speech, symphonies, and plays. "I like to read. I picked up a lot of good language habits from reading. I learned to diagram sentences in school, and I am still very good at it." Her best friend is an English teacher; sometimes they communicate and one says, "That has to be the run-on sentence of all run-on sentences. Who picks up on that?" All of this background is to explain why she has become a valued and trusted friend.

Back in 2011, Irene tried to take a step and her legs would not move. "That changed everything." She was diagnosed with a slipped disk in her lower vertebra causing numbness and weakness in her legs. She had four corrective surgical attempts to alleviate the problems. She related that the eighteen days in physical therapy at the Fort Worth hospital taught her to transfer with a transfer board, which was very helpful. She was catheterized during surgery to simplify bathroom problems, which caused its own complications. Irene was very weak and uncoordinated in her upper body, had poor fine motor skills, and near total paralysis in her legs. She could not stand on her own, but they used a standing frame which helped a lot. They trained her upper body with arm-crank exercise but did no work on her lower body. At that point, she could not feed herself without spilling it all down her front. She was transferred directly to a Stephenville nursing facility, which totally exhausted her.

She was mobile only in a wheelchair with someone pushing her; there was no mobility independence. She could not get from the bed to the rolling table, bathroom, or anywhere. She could not turn herself over in bed; she could not pick up anything from the floor if she dropped it from the wheelchair. Irene's perception was that "they didn't know what to do with me. There was contention between the therapists and the rest of the staff. They got me up at six or seven o'clock in the morning, and I was in the chair until seven o'clock at night." She had speech therapy which "really got my brain in gear—that was *really* important." Irene spent one hundred days, which was all that Medicare and insurance would pay. She wore the catheter for another seventy days; it was removed when she still had thirty days in the nursing home. They used a standing frame and allowed her to read from the upright position, which was good for her brain development. She was discharged to her home, where a home-health nurse and her husband teamed up to provide care. It was a good experience which helped her gain some independence, sharing with the cooking chores like chopping vegetables from her wheelchair.

In September 2014, Irene found the LWMB when current client David and his dad Duane passed the information along to Irene. They constantly encouraged each other at church. After her training began in the LWMB, in her fluent reflection, she said, "I had been feeling alone, left-out, and isolated. Depression that I fought all my life, but now this was *real* depression. The only person I talked to was my husband. Here I found a community where I was immediately accepted. Most of us here have come from a long journey to get here. We've been through months and months of therapy and been told numerous times that we can't do that. I came from not being able to move a big toe to walking with a walker, from not being able to open a carton of Half-and-Half or cutting a piece of meat. I still can't jab the meat with a fork, but we're not through training yet either. I brought my tweezers today so I can learn how to use those again." (Sohm 2015)

Irene is so well spoken, it is really easy to transcribe her conversations because she talks in complete sentences, has a charming vocabulary, and communicates beautifully. As I value Irene's feedback from her hours in the LWMB, I asked how the trainers are doing, to which she explains that anyone of fifteen trainers are "totally amazing. I can't wait to get here. They have exceeded expectations from the fall semester [immediate past], totally dedicated, willing to try almost anything, to help me with flexibility, strength, and endurance. The emotional support here in the LWMB is outstanding. Getting to know each other makes it personal and personable. For instance, I'd like to be able to walk from the couch to the kitchen without my walker, so I share this goal with my trainers, and we work toward that goal. As a result, last week I walked seven times—that's seven times up and back without holding onto anything. I'm less frightened here. At the nursing home, they're constantly cautioning against falling. Here in the LWMB, if I were to fall, I'm not falling very far because they're always there."

Justifying our existence and our pre-professional staff, Irene comments, "It's like going to the beauty college. Somebody has to practice on somebody." I asked Irene how our program effects depression. "I don't have any," she quickly exclaimed. "When I'm done in here, I miss the people and the involvement. Interaction with other people is critical."

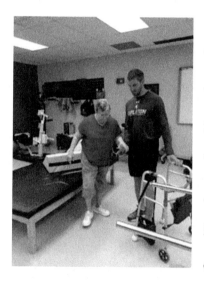

In March 2015 Irene said, "It's really nice for trainers to think about you. I carried them in my head during spring break. They think outside the room." As we watched several trainers in a group, not yet focused on client training, "There's nothing like having fun at work," she said approvingly. I almost forget that during her casual dialogues, she completed over 156,000 steps covering 86 miles on the NuStep. I stood by her during one of her prescribed Technogym UBE training sessions. During the summer and fall training sessions, she completed 15 workouts on the UBE totaling over 4.5 hours and covering 56km. She commented, "You hardly know you're working out. With somebody standing beside me talking and learning about me and me learning about them, it's easy. You don't pay extra for caring. They do this because that's who they are–student interns. Nick never fails to say something to me that I take home in my head."

What a nice testimony for our LWMB Interns. Knowing that those interns were only there another five weeks, I asked Irene, "How am I going to find more interns like these?"

"Oh, they will find you," she said intuitively.

Irene had good news from her cardiologist; her blood pressure was excellent. She reported that working out there, along with increases in vegetables in the diet, helped significantly. In addition to the cardiovascular improvements, the regular exercise was definitely helping her mobility. She was able to help her husband more in cooking chores. One morning she was up early. "I fixed my hair with my right hand," noting that that had not been possible for 3.5 years since the paralysis. "I had no trouble getting into and out of the truck, about eight times yesterday, and I am accomplishing more domestic chores than ever." According to Irene, those improvements were directly related to her activities in the LWMB, motivated by the student interns. Her transition from wheelchair to walker to kitchen to truck, etc., presented problems, and we would address them specifically in her training activities. Irene also prepared a corn beef dish for the cooker one morning (while standing) prior to coming to work out. Irene was getting more involved in church and other civic activities. "My brain is working better for sure. I had a bit of an emotional setback last Friday that I struggled with all weekend. Before, it would have sent me to the mental hospital," she noted candidly.

Remember Irene's wish to be able to use tweezers again? Student-interns Julia and Colton added some exercises with hand weights to her routine. By the end of the first week, she was already able to use tweezers and open a jar of pickles in the kitchen. She credited the kinesiology team with knowing what she did last workout and planning for that day accordingly. She referred to that, in her usual intellectual analysis, as "unintended consequences of working with hand weights.

Why did this make my hands stronger? I'm just holding onto the blooming things… and my handwriting has improved to the point where I'm not ashamed of it." The trainers admitted frankly that they really had not foreseen the training benefits extending to handwriting and opening a jar of pickles.

You could see that Irene had made a huge impression on all of us. I tried to record her at various times in our conversations, anticipating more jewels of wisdom. During one such occasion, Irene identified student trainers with whom she had developed a two-way confidence. She was able to confide in them, knowing they have her best interest at stake. "They have such varied backgrounds, different plans." I asked Irene to describe the clients that came here for training day in and day out. "They come here with smiles on their faces in spite of their difficult challenges." She preferred that instead of what I sometimes described as problems. "The unconditional love encountered in here changes people," adding, "forever." What a tribute to a group of unselfish trainers.

Given the nice rally to that point, I asked her about her goals. "My husband expects me to walk across the room and help in the garden." My thought was that it seemed reasonable. Irene exclaimed, "That's not going to happen." I said defiantly, "You don't think we can get you there?" She quickly added, "I don't want to go to the garden." Oh, I see. We have discovered a character worthy of a book.

Joel—Paraplegia

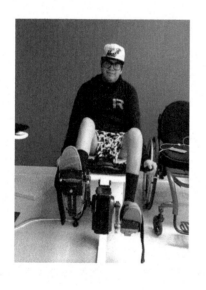

In June 2014 the twenty-two-year-old young man drove his pickup without his seatbelt to his friend's house. On a rainy day, Joel's truck hydroplaned unexpectedly, ending upside down in the ditch. A friend pulled him out and ran for help, but the T11–T12 spinal cord injury caused immediate paralysis of his legs.

After four hours of stabilizing vital signs at a local hospital, he was transferred to a metroplex hospital in Fort Worth. He stayed there for one week before being taken back to his hometown where he trained two days per week with a local physical therapist. Three assistants worked with him on his gait although he had no muscle tone or stability in the hips, knees, and ankles. Joel could accomplish no voluntary movements with his legs, so all of the leg movements in the walker were assisted. Little effort was directed to gaining basic strength in preparation for gait training. Upon his release, he was independently mobile only in his wheel chair.

October 2014 was the beginning of Joel's rookie season in the LWMB, which he described as a "good place to come,. good environment and people to help you out. It's a motivating thing. Thanks for letting me come." His trainers were very systematic in his use of the NuStep devices. They initially used the lateral supports for his legs because he still had no leg control. These devices braced his knees during the bilateral arm and leg stepping motion. Joel's strong upper body provided all the power for the initial training while his legs moved passively. He was able to maintain rhythmic motion for three thousand steps in thirty-five minutes per session. Over three semesters his diligence became apparent as he completed 92,500 arm and leg steps covering 51 miles, averaging 2862 steps and 1.6 miles per training session.

His trainers gravitated his workouts to the Psycle where at first he could not generate the two pounds of force necessary to power the pedals. Adapting that exercise attempt, the trainers set the left crank arm in the perfect position on top of the rotation where he soon learned to move the left pedal an inch or two. Trainers then moved the right pedal to top position where he could, with great difficulty, move the crank arm slightly although by his own admission not with his legs. After those very fatiguing attempts, he pushed arms on legs to produce continuous leg motions, gradually working up to one thousand revolutions per session. In six weeks, he was still unable to accomplish independent leg pedaling. Three months later on January 16, 2015, Joel did his first revolution on the Psycle with no hands.

Five months after his arrival in the LWMB, he stopped using lateral supports during three thousand steps on the NuStep and did three unassisted revolutions on the Psycle, which he said takes all the force he can generate from his core muscles. He still had little sensation or active control of his legs during cycling. His own motivation was exceptional, and the encouragement from trainers was vital as he continued to increase his unassisted leg cycling record.

Flash forward one year from his first workout, I walked into the lab from class where I saw Joel pedaling backward, rather casually against five pounds of electromagnetic resistance on the Psycle for three hundred legs-only revolutions. "This is my favorite workout where I can work by myself pushing the pedals." On that same day, he said he stood unassisted and balanced in the parallel bars for ten minutes.

January 2016, Joel remembered that he could not pedal at all, and he was able to pedal with his legs alone. "Now I try to do four hundred revolutions forward and four hundred backward with legs alone."

After all this success, I asked Joel, "What's the secret to your continued improvement?"

He said, "Not giving up, working hard, and attitude is everything."

"What's your goal for this semester?" I asked.

He quickly responded, "Walk by June, I've got a big wedding to go to." Student-intern Sammie said, "We've got to do this piece by piece, and we're going to do everything we can do to help you to that goal" (Chavez 2016).

The following quote came from LWMB Supervisor Elizabeth who posted a report on a very insightful visit with Joel. It is particularly revealing as it represents two youngsters developing a genuine and caring relationship.

> I had the chance to sit down and talk to Joel about his injury, goals, and Stephen Hawking. He seems like a shy person and he is, but once you get to know him and talk to him he really begins to open up. He talked to me about his injury, which was an incom-

plete spinal cord injury. When he first came into the lab he was only able to move his toes, and well now he's able to move most of his body. He sure has come a long way, he has gained so much strength and confidence. We talked about our goals and what our future might hold. He tells me that he leaves motivational quotes all over the place in his room. His goals are to walk by the end of the year, enroll at Tarleton, and become a physical therapist to help young adults who are going through what he is and to be a motivational speaker. (Cisneros, Google+ 2015)

The takeaway here is that with a personal relationship and supervised training extended beyond conventional health care, a rally in wellness and motor behavior, even an attitude can be expected. This translates into hope, greater independence, and personal expectations.

Jeffery—Spinal Surgery/Paralysis

Jeffery was diagnosed in February 2015 with a spinal infection that degenerated four of his thoracic vertebrae. On the second surgery, the surgeons installed rods to stabilize that part of the vertebral column. Rehabilitation efforts lasted about three weeks, during which time he worked up to ten minutes per session on arm and leg movements. He was released from rehabilitation confined to a wheelchair as he had lost his ability to stand and had little control of his legs.

As a former FedEx delivery man living in a nearby town, his decision to move to Stephenville in April 2015 was based upon having access to training in the LWMB. In his rookie season with us, he started training with us in April of 2015. Student-interns supervised his initial activities on the NuStep. Unable to move his legs, Jeffery was able to accomplish low-intensity, rhythmic movements with his arms and legs. Training sessions varied from twenty to forty minutes of continuous movements. In seven months, he accomplished seventy thousand steps and thirty-eight miles, averaging two thousand two hundred steps and over a mile per training session.

Gradually, his trainers encouraged more activity, usually lasting over two hours. One of his favorite workouts was on the Psycle, which allowed continuous leg cycling using only power from his legs. Initial efforts at independent leg cycling were very painful, so trainers set the crank arms in hole number 1, which is a crank radius of 27 mm (about one inch). This short range of motion made the knee pain tolerable and required about a six-pound force alternately from each leg in order to produce independent and continuous movement. The direct-drive energy regeneration flywheel feature of the Psycle was effective in keeping the pedals moving between power strokes.

In a period of six sessions on the Psycle, Jeffery was able to tolerate a longer range of motion in hole number 2 (about one inch longer in crank radius). Although the pain was intense again, he had confidence that it would again subside with each training session. Skip forward eight more weeks and Jeffery completed one thousand revolutions in crank arm number 6. With each progressive one-inch crank arm incre-ment, the story was the same: pain returned and diminished with subsequent training sessions. The progression continued to the fall 2015 semester when he often completed over two thousand five hundred revolutions per session on the Psycle, accumulating over fifty-two thousand revolutions in twen-ty-four hours of training for the year. He looked forward to completing a full range of motion in hole number 7, enabling greater freedom and strength of movement.

After five weeks in the LWMB, trainers Chris and Colton moved him to the parallel bars, where Jeffery practiced stand-ing where most of the required force was produced from his arms. Initially, he elevated and stood using mostly the force from the arms. As he stood, he tried with each session to bear more weight on his legs. Stepping within the parallel bars was then attempted, with Jeffery able to complete more and more trips up and down the bars. "My best workout was twen-ty-nine minutes of continuous walking with only occasional use of my hands for balance," according to Jeffery.

After several sessions in the parallel bars, trainers then accompanied Jeffery to the kinesiology base path. Using his walker, trainers timed his initial trip around the diamond (440 feet (134.1 m) at 13:50, including one resting period. Then progressively over the next few weeks, his times decreased to six minutes with no resting periods. As the lab is not open during weekends, Jeffery started supplementing his walking in the local park, which included some elevation changes that added a new dimension to his efforts. He graduated from there to using two canes instead of his walker, completing a current record of 0.85 mile. Jeffery has begun to practice on the kinesiology base path, taking the weight off one cane for a few steps at a time. He hoped to graduate to one cane soon.

At the time of writing this, Jeffery has trained progressively with three different groups of student interns—spring 2014, summer 2014, and fall 2015 with each group picking up where the previous group ended. That's the nature of the kinesiology team; even as one group graduates, their understudies are ready, willing, and able to assume progressive training as long as he needs it. As Jeffery reflected back on his first eight months in the LWMB, his interpretation of his progress is telling, "I left conventional care on a Thursday in April, and on Monday of the next week, I had moved my home to here and begun training with you. If I had gone home instead, I think my depression would have progressed to the point where I might not have been able to recover. Even when I began training here, I would go home, and when no one was home with me, I became dis-couraged between workouts. The lowest part of my day was at home and alone, but as I began to improve, the anticipation of the next lab session provided me enough motivation to ward off my depression."

In response to my question about his future goals, he

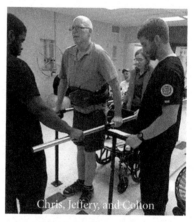

Chris, Jeffery, and Colton

After weeks of training on the NuStep, the Psycle, and the OrthoSys, Jeffery attempted standing in the parallel bars with wife Peggy behind with the wheelchair. For months, he wore his five-inch belt for abdominal stability.

replied, "I'd like to be in better health than before my paralysis. I want to walk easily and return to work." Jeffery's desire is to get back in the game. We at the LWMB need no more gratification than this.

After LWMB?

At the time of writing this, the previous featured clients in this book are still actively engaged in supervised training in the LWMB, so their stories are not complete. They are quite literally works in progress as they continue to strive for improvements in wellness and motor behavior. They typically appreciate their new active lifestyle and understand some of the many beneficial side-effects. Through the years, many have left our supervised training and continue physical activities at home or in conventional fitness facilities. Such is the case of the following characters:

At seventy years of age and knowing little about our program, Ed and I visited about a recent newspaper article covering a LWMB client. He mentioned that his back had hurt for probably ten years. I asked what the problem was, to which he responded, "Oh, I'm just old."

I said to him, "Your back is not supposed to hurt, why not come in and work with us for a while?" His son, a local physician agreed and wrote his clearance to train with us. He joined the team, and the trainers suggested rather leisurely rides on the Psycle.

After four weeks (three sessions per week) of the low-intensity, rhythmic leg cycling, Ed came into my office and said, "We need to talk." Of course that's what we do a lot of. He said he had awakened at two o'clock that morning.

"Okay," I said, thinking, "Where is this going?"

Ed continued, "My back didn't hurt." This was the first time in many years that he was pain-free, evidence that exercise is medicine.

Gail joined our program after years of arthritis had damaged the joint until the right knee was replaced. Conventional post-surgical physical therapy provided her little improvement. "There I was placed on a regular bike, not a recumbent like yours, for probably five minutes of warm up. It never increased for the ten weeks of my therapy. They didn't do near what you do here." She began training in the LWMB and reported that "you pushed me farther, gave me more of what I needed, and I can tell the difference." Gail gave all the credit to the trainers in the LWMB, but a glance at her training habits tells the rest of the story. During the summer semester, she took advantage of the opportunities to train, accomplishing over forty thousand arm and leg steps, over twenty-two machine-calculated miles on the NuStep. During that semester and the subsequent fall 2015 semester, she added 60,500 revolutions on the Psycle in over 21 hours of training. Did I mention that she is past seventy years old? She said of her diligent efforts, "I enjoy coming here. The trainers are great. I want to train to avoid the other knee replacement. Your students are enthusiastic. They bounce off you." Thanks for the vote of confidence.

Paul was a seventy-two-year-old who coached NCAA basketball for the love of the game and who hardly recognized his five hundred wins. After retiring from forty years of coaching, he became increasingly aware of shoulder pain that continued to progress until he could no longer swing a golf club. He said, "Now golf's the one thing I do that keeps me going." His orthopedic specialist's MRI confirmed damage that was going to require surgery, which was scheduled for the month of July. In order to get strong for surgery, he participated in twelve low-intensity strategic training sessions in the LWMB, after which he called to cancel his appointment for shoulder surgery. He accompanied his wife and her kinesiology class on a June international kinesiology field course in Scotland, where he played, with no shoulder pain, twelve rounds of golf on one of the oldest golf courses in the world. Furthermore, walking ten rounds of golf pulling a cart was excellent exercise for his artificial hip and knee.

Paul attributes the spark that started his rally to the student-interns and the strategic training activities in the LWMB. They got him on base, and I'm pretty sure that Paul just stole second, sliding head first under the tag. However, simple and surprising the kinesiology team played the role of The Deacon in Holmes's poem designing the perfect organism. The "weakest part mus' stan' the strain." They fixed the shoulder and made it "uz strong uz the rest."

Upon his return to the US, Paul continued a similar regime of exercises at home in his garage, using rubber bands for variable resistance. At the time of writing this, he teaches golf at the university and continues to be a pain-free avid golfer. The takeaway here is to give strategic exercise a chance to produce adaptive healing. By the way, Paul found a way to put his renewed health and incredible coaching talent to work—he just won an area championship with a team of ten-year-old boys. How much is that worth?

In March 2014 at age twenty-five, Chelsea rolled her truck and experienced a broken neck with paralysis of her right arm and hand. After surgery, she was in a halo (a device to stabilize the head and neck) during four weeks of intensive care plus four weeks of inpatient rehabilitation. She walked in her room with a walker and trained with PT, OT, and ST three hours per day. The halo was removed in June 2014 when she returned home and continued training at a local rehabilitation facility. Chelsea's progress was slow but stopped in August, like so many others, when the insurance coverage was exhausted.

Still unable to train independently in September 2014, she commuted thirty round-trip miles to the LWMB for supervised training. She described her trainers as "amazing, they work with you and want all of us to do the best we can." Her activities included continuous rhythmic exercises on the NuStep, ExN'Flex, and Technogym UBE while standing, along with creative activities for balance and coordination. The sessions lasted 2.5 to 3 hours per day and three days per week. The extended training opportunity was critical to Chelsea's independence. By December 2014, her improved wellness and motor behavior gave her the confidence "to go home and incorporate this into my daily activities." She anticipated that "it's not going to be easy. The body reverts to the easiest way. I'm not sure how long I can keep it up." Her compliments to the LWMB activities:

I would recommend this lab to anybody who wants to improve. For instance, in local conventional rehabilitation I trained 30 minutes on my arm and went home. At LWMB, we worked on the arm, but also the rest of the body and "wellness as a whole." We worked on balance. Making friends was just as important—meeting others who understand your problem. People you can relate to; Clarence is my inspiration. Every time I see [client] Brandi standing up in the OrthoSys, I tear up, because I grew up with her. I remember her playing basketball. This would not be possible without the LWMB. It's easy to give up every day. (Johnson 2014)

At the time of writing this, Chelsea was back home, employed, and maintained her health; we celebrate her victory.

As an outstanding athlete, Kurt Gross played collegiate football at Trinity University. He sustained a neck injury in a car wreck that resulted in quadriplegia. He chose to continue his education here and train in the LWMB. He learned to accomplish unassisted leg cycling using the Psycle which he pedaled from his motorized wheelchair. He said the three training years from 1999–2002 were "the healthiest I have been throughout my post-injury years." He stayed physically active while he finished his bachelor's degree. Highly success-ful in academics, he completed his jurisprudence doctorate at the University of Texas. He and Shelly, his wife of sixteen years have three sons. Dr. Gross became a Houston-based attorney, practicing in the area of oil and gas (Gross 2016).

A potentially catastrophic accident took Dean out of a faculty position at our university. He was in hospital intensive care for three months and in a coma for one month. After months of rehabilitation efforts, Dean showed some signs of improvement. His wife Barbara and his physical therapist, Frank, accompanied him to the LWMB where collaborative efforts expanded his training regimen. The NuStep train-ing was very beneficial as his exercise endurance gradually improved; cumulative training included eight hours and twenty-nine thousand steps covering over sixteen miles. As the trust grew and the insurance money ran out, he came unaccompanied to the LWMB.

Dean then graduated to the Psycle, where he spent many hours regaining his mobility. His jovial personality entertained the trainers and fellow clients. As fellow professors, we shared many refreshing stories about student and university progress, to which we were both committed. His communication skills were brilliant and obvious. I knew it was just a matter of time before he would be able to return to his university service.

On June 4, 2014, I was visiting with a new client. In the middle of the conversation, I saw a figure out of the corner of my eye who walked in and his six-foot-three-inch body looked seven feet tall, standing up straight in a bright yellow shirt. He looked around the lab as if to locate somebody to pick on and joke

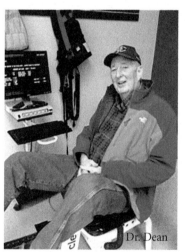

Dr. Dean trained on the NuStep three days per week, here on the Psycle.

with. A striking figure, I went over to greet him and to congratulate him on his recovery and his appearance. I said to him, "Welcome back," and he thought I meant welcome back to the lab for summer training, but what I really meant was "Welcome back to the faculty." Coming from his near catatonic state to full function was amazing and inspirational. To the casual observer, it might appear that he recovered spontaneously—they didn't see how far his injuries had set him back. They didn't see the hours and hours of training that he accomplished in the LWMB. It is certainly a thrill to have him back on full-time faculty status.

Outside the June 5 morning, Clarence was sitting outside after his workout, waiting for Linda to pick him up about noon. Dr. Dean was walking by on his way out. In his jovial style, he said to Clarence, "Looking good, Clarence" as she leaned over and shook his hand. He walked over to me and qualified my compliment, "Looking pretty good, Dr. Priest" and laughed.

View from the Bleachers—Perspectives of Fellow Faculty

Dr. Tom Tallach. Upon joining the Tarleton Kinesiology faculty in 2013, I was only mildly familiar with Dr. Priest's work and the Lab for Wellness and Motor Behavior (LWMB). My first semester, our departmental circumstances required that I teach a class on adapted physical activity that included programming for individuals with disabilities. Having spent the prior twenty years in college athletics as a coach and administrator, I considered this the epitome of playing out of position. Nonetheless, I was a rookie and confident that I could teach anything with just a little more knowledge than the students in front of me. But how would

I add visual and experiential elements to the class to enhance its appeal, you know make it more interesting? Well, necessity is in fact the mother of invention, and in my case, it was the mother of figuring out what the heck to do. I quickly came to the realization that I had access to a practitioner in the very field, and his office was right down the hall. There was no doubt in my mind that the LWMB would fit like a well-oiled glove in terms of helping students learn how to help the special population. However, my presumptions about how that would happen were completely wrong.

Planning class visits to the LWMB gave me the occasion to learn more about both the program and its founder and facilitator. Listening to Dr. Priest in one-on-one office visits as well as his addressing students in my classes, my eyes were opened not only in regard to the health-care challenges faced by so many of the clients but also to what makes our program here so successful. As expected, my students and I did learn about what it took to serve the clientele, but it wasn't so much technical knowledge. It's more about a certain mindset. A ball player might call it a feel for the game. It's understanding that life goes on regardless of the capabilities of one's neuromuscular system and so does the pursuit of happiness and independence, the desire to be challenged and to achieve, and the desire to develop life-giving relationships. Recognizing and helping people meet these needs in a physical fitness context with a little knowledge and a ton of creativity is what happens here. It's also about problem solving and refusing to believe that we can't find a way. I now know what my more-experienced faculty colleagues knew all along. I wasn't playing out of position after all.

This program is the embodiment of our institutional core value of service and our strategic goal of student engagement. It is exactly what we say we want to do. It works beautifully for us. For me, however, feeling good about what we do here isn't enough. The demand is out there. (Not surprisingly I suppose as there's always a demand for things that are good and free.) The problem solver in me wants to know why more organizations can't create the same type of synergistic enterprise. As a university, we have an advantage because learning and service are products and have tangible value in this context. Certainly, other colleges and universities could do this as many seek opportunities for students to engage in service learning. But what other types of organizations could benefit from such an enterprise and how? While many hospital therapy units may not benefit from state support and student tuition to balance their budgets, many do benefit from gifts and grants, and this is a cause worthy of philanthropic support. Many hospitals are in competitive markets and need to distinguish themselves as community servants. There always seems to be cash in the marketing and public relations budget to sponsor a worthwhile event or purchase print advertising. With a little creativity, here's an opportunity to make a real impact using existing assets (no cash). That's a home run! Many hospitals that are not in competitive markets benefit from public support and can benefit similarly by demonstrating good stewardship of that support. In either case, the clients of course win; student volunteers win by gaining experience, and the organization wins by demonstrating the willingness to give back to the community and in a way that is cost effective. There are so many who could benefit and we have the game plan right here. Let's play ball!

Dr. Jarrod Schenewark. For nearly twenty years, Dr. Priest has labored to restore function and life to bodies bent and broken by disease and injury. He opened up the doors of a public university in order to heal a segment of the public with no place to go. And he has done so by using the knowledge found in the discipline of kinesiology.

The Hall of Fame catcher and amateur philosopher, Yogi Berra, is credited with saying, "You can observe a lot by just watching." There is much truth in that quote, for I have observed confidence rekindled, dignity restored, and knowledge resurrected through applied exercise at the Lab for Wellness and Motor Behavior (LWMB).

The labor which Dr. Priest manages focuses on the body. However, the work has a great impact on the spirit and the mind. When I see the individuals for whom the lab is designed to serve I see individuals with confidence. They have confidence that they will not be the indigent, dependent, and unproductive community members that society often assumes individuals with similar disorders will become. The flame of confidence not only is rekindled in the clients but also in the many student workers.

The lab is not only designed for service to the injured but also for the enhancement of the student workers. As I have visited the lab, I find the students working there to be among the brightest and most enthusiastic students I have encountered. This is saying a lot as I have had the opportunity to work with students at the University of California, Berkeley, and the University of Texas in Austin, which are two of the premier public universities in the world. The students working in the lab are not only in a field but on the field. The confidence of students in their own ability and in the transformative power of all which makes up the discipline of kinesiology impacts the lives of those with whom the students work.

This confidence gained by students and clients, I believe, converts into dignity. As the students who work in the lab walk across the campus they hold their heads high as individuals deserving of respect. They are involved in a great work similar to the students found in nursing or in ROTC, which is the giving of themselves, their time, talent, and energy in the service of others.

Poise, pride, self-possession are restored to clients who were told that they were no longer welcomed by other organizations whether for a belief they could not be helped or for the lack of ability to pay for further treatment.

The work of Dr. Priest and the LWMB is significant because it helps resurrect knowledge from the field of kinesiology (formerly known as physical education) that people can be helped through the use of exercise that the field of kinesiology is much more than fun, games, and sport.

The ancient physician Herodicus believed that exercise was "just as important to provide against disease in the healthy body as it is to cure him who is already attacked" (Berryman 1992). While much research has been done on the disease preventative nature of exercise, Herodicus's statement sheds light on the nature of Dr. Priest's lab's work that exercise can cure disease.

Likewise, similar concepts were put forth in John Pugh's *Physiological, Theoretic, and Practical Treatise on the Utility of the Service of Muscular Action for Restoring the Power of the Limbs* (1794). Within his book, Pugh dedicated a chapter on the necessity and importance of exercise in order to bring back useful function to disabled limbs. Pugh's work also contained support for therapeutic exercise from the ancient doctors Hippocrates, Galen, and Medieval Venetian nobleman Cornaro (Berryman and Park, 1992).

Finally, when I see the work of the lab, I think of the outstanding work performed by R. Tait McKenzie, one of the most notable leaders of our profession (Gerber 1971). McKenzie sought the treatment of patients with physical disabilities and focused on the importance of individual improvements through exercise. McKenzie based his work on previous physical educators, such as Archibald McLaren, Per Henrik Ling, and the Swedish Gymnastic System as well as the work of machines and pulley weights of the system put forth by Dudley Allen Sargent. During and following the First World War, McKenzie used his knowledge of those systems to devise a new system to modified regular exercise and developed special exercise for those convalescing. He used exercise in order to "reeducate control and strength" in individuals who had lost them through neglect, injury, or "enforced idleness of hospital life" (Mason 2008).

Roberta Park, who has spent a lifetime studying the history of our field, lamented that "we lag behind in translating science into practice" (Park 2008). From my observations, this is not the case with Dr. Joe Priest and the Lab for Wellness and Motor Behavior. The lab has blessed many lives including the clients, students, and a host of family members. The work connects our field to the past while at the same time showing our way into the future. It is my hope that the efforts of Dr. Priest will be recognized and duplicated.

View from First-Base—
Perspectives of a Hospital
Administrator

 A common thought in the current health care system is that care begins at first base in the hospital

or at the physician's office. Too often, however, this becomes

a system that takes care of disease—a disease-care system.

As president and hospital administrator, Chris spoke with

great understanding of the challenges facing acute care in

his hospital as well as in our American health-care system.

He said that health care providers are necessarily expanding

their perspective to what he suggested is the new continuum

of care. In this model, health care begins in the home, in

communities, and in jobs, where people are attentive to their own health. They assume active roles in their own health and wellness. They take advantage of what is known to be a powerful force in maintaining health—that exercise is medicine. After the patient's treatment and release from the hospital, Chris described it, "We're looking more broadly at extending health care beyond our walls. Hospital inpatient readmissions have become critical as Medicare does not reimburse for these services. We're trying to do things to help insure that patients don't have to come back. Your university program has the potential effect of reducing the chances of return visits to the hospital or emergency room. Even in patients with many comorbid conditions, the work that you're doing with them physically and emotionally would have a very positive impact on other issues such as skin wounds, cardiorespiratory and pulmonary health. Family members and other caregivers would also be the beneficiaries of this improved patient wellness."

Chris sees the prospect of extending health care to an evidence-based practice.

We're willing to do things that effectively reduce readmission. If your program can help accomplish this, then as an administrator, even as a tax payer, I am interested. We all win when downstream medical expenses are cut or eliminated through decreased use of drugs and services. A reduction in the patient's dependence on prescription drugs would have a huge downstream cost impact on the overall health care system as well as the obvious benefit for the patient. As we strive to improve our health care models, maybe this is something we can consider as a viable extension of care. The best practices model evolves from evidence that something really works. Maybe there are some opportunities here to improve our continuum of care. (Leu 2016)

For twenty years this extended care is about all client Jerry needed. After his release from conventional care, he took advantage of an opportunity at the LWMB where sixty successive kinesiology teams delivered movement activities to ease his pain. We all win when his extraordinary health virtually eliminated downstream medical expenses. He got a chance to score and win given a free pass—an intentional walk. His teammates in the LWMB are willing to sacrifice in order to get him around the bases. They'll bunt or hit behind the runner even risking their own demise. Jerry and Clarence and Rickie and Randy provide evidence that *after everybody else gave up*, relentless commitment to our movement model contributes to their independence and wellness. Their payback to society is their acquired wellness, their independence, their disuse of health care services. Remember Bill who trained in the LWMB, got well and returned to work after his stroke, and became the number 1 commercial real estate salesman in the county—two years running. What's that worth to American health care?

You can't score if you don't get past first base.

View from the Dugout—
Perspectives of a Key
Physician

 A practicing physician for thirty years, Neal had a stroke in 2010. The stroke caused paralysis of his left arm and leg, and he had great difficulty standing and walking. In California, Neal found a therapist and educator whom he liked, an immigrant from Bagdad, Waleed Al-Oboudi (Neuro-INFRAH Center, La Jolla, California), who uses unconventional treatment methods and tools. He administers excellent and innovative therapy and provides education and equipment for the therapeutic community. Much of Neal's joint flexibility now is attributed to this early treatment.

In December 2014, Neal started commuting seventy miles round trip to train with us. It was apparent that we could help him with our supervised low-intensity, high-repetition movements. The payback was immediate; his perspective is invaluable: "I have dealt with the hopelessness that I feel when I can't be a physician anymore, yet I know I have a lot of knowledge that can help others. I want to start branching out, using my intelligence and skills to help others. One of the things I love about being here [in the LWMB] is helping students develop pathways of compassion and feelings. They watch people like me get better—by coming in here together, we're all healed—your students and those of us who come because of our disability."

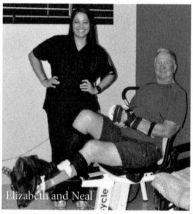

Elizabeth and Neal

Training on the Psycle included 30-45 minutes, completing 1,500 revolutions per session. Crank arm lengths were adjusted to one of seven motion ranges.

Neal's contributions to us continued as he shared his amazing insight into the art of healing, attitudinal healing for individuals with severe transforming illnesses or events such as spinal injury or strokes.

These transforming events cause changes in the body that are not easily reversed. You easily get depressed and suicidal; therefore, rehabilitation has to be transformative in the mind. You have to take the opportunity to transform your mind in face of devastating changes in the body. Communicating these ideas is vital. (Sutherland 2015)

In our one-on-one conversation, Neal's gratitude was direct: "Thanks for giving me the opportunity to express my feelings. They've been inside me for a long time, and for me to express them is healing. And seeing your positive response to me makes me feel even more empowered. We are a team together—the LWMB is all about teamwork."

The student-interns in the LWMB immediately befriended him and enjoyed supervising his training. During his 2015 training sessions on the NuStep, he completed over

42,000 steps and 23 miles, averaging 2,200 steps and 1.2 miles per session. The exercise on the NuStep allowed Neal to experience rhythmic movement against a low resistance, which he easily endured for twenty-five to thirty minutes. After the warm up on the NuStep, Neal walked with assistance across the clubhouse to the Psycle, which provided him another opportunity to exercise continuously and independently. Neal typically completed one thousand revolutions forward and five hundred backward per session and again at a low-intensity; he was able to maintain rhythmic movement with his legs. During both of these exercises, the power for continuous movement was provided mostly by his right side which was unaffected by the stroke. The passive movement of the left side provided a training stimulus for paralyzed muscles affected by the stroke. This ability to do independent exercise had great significance; it allowed Neal to feel successful. He said, "It feels good to do something and see that I am the one doing it, not somebody doing it for me."

The Technogym UBE (Technogym, USA Corp, Fairfield, New Jersey) allowed for more independent exercise utilizing the normal power of his strong side to power continuous movement of his paralyzed arm. The benefits of moving paralyzed muscles were verified prior to 2000 (D. S. Willoughby) and 2002 (D. S. Willoughby).

These exercise routines prepared Neal for practicing his walking gait. Remember graduate assistant Chris? He was the trainer who I implied could bench press the building, having completed his NCAA football eligibility at 375 pounds. His presence gave Neal the confidence to begin walking with a cane around the kinesiology base path. After a year of training, I witnessed him and Chris walking up and down the kinesiology stairs, much to his/our celebration. Some of Neal's off-the-cuff interpretations were priceless:

This lab gives young, impressionable kids an opportunity to experience the joy that comes with having compassion towards another. They end up doing a whole lot out of their desire to better serve another human. They use their knowledge base, the things they've learned here, to practice compassion. It's not a curricular item, but it comes with the LWMB territory, and given that stimuli [our Applied Learning Experience- my words], these bright, young, generally athletic kids want to assist others in regaining the joy of mobility... just their presence helps.

Neal continued his insightful interpretation of the LWMB:

The lab is a blending of exercise and wellness. Being in the lab is a choice for all who are there. Students volunteer; those of us with motor dysfunction come with wellness at our core. People are built to move. When we move we get our needs met; we feel better. Feeling better engenders hope, and the base of wellness is hope. Hope shared between students and clients creates bonds of compassion, friendship, and improvement in the exercise experience. We all improve from within and without, we share and encourage. I am greeted each morning at the lab with "What would you like to do today," and the implied reality is "I will help you. Let's get started!" Together much more is achieved. Trust develops, strength improves, and movement becomes easier. Life looks brighter—wellness is felt. Frustration retreats to the back of our minds. We see and feel hope!

Thank you, Dr. Neal. May you experience the inner peace that comes from knowing that your words are curative.

Conclusion

	1	2	3	4	5	6	7	8	9	R	H	E
CUBS	0	1	1	02	4	0				8	9	5
Home	0	0	0	0	0	0				0	3	4

There is little dignity in loss of health after retirement or before. The LWMB model illustrates how dignity can be attained and maintained after retirement by engaging in a relentless training program.

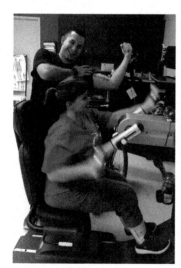

Training in the LWMB is relentless as long as the clients need adaptive training. It is unaffected by fees or insurance payments, and it can continue indefinitely.

Trainer Blake, who became a commissioned Officer in the United States Army, and client Kristin work on the Technogym Upper-Body ergometer.

The stories of what can be accomplished after being released from the health care system are meaningful. What is not being accomplished in weeks of conventional therapy may be realized in response to years of supervised training. *After everybody else gave up*, a glimpse of hope returns as clients enter a long-term contract for major-league recovery of wellness and motor behavior. The inviting, positive, accepting, and attentive environment prevails and dignity may be gained in the experience. Could it be that as Thomas suggested in 1979 that we have learned a method to cope effectively with most chronic diseases?

A veteran of four consecutive semesters of service in the LWMB, Shelana said to me, "With your guidance, I was able to discover my passion for helping others. You have me hooked for life! This lab has changed the lives of lots of people, including myself."

After ten weeks of service in the LWMB, student-intern Emily submitted:

Every day I get to go into the lab and see all of these things happening just makes me want to push myself even harder to figure out a way to open one of these... I have made it my life goal to one day be able to open a clinic like the lab and help people in the same situations. (Stock, Google+ 2015)

Implementation of this simple and extended health-care model at other American universities is feasible. Existing agencies, including the aforementioned NSA, ASIA, UCP, NMSS, AF, and SBA are already funded for the education required to operationalize such a plan. Our supervised activity program can provide hope for currently underserved specific populations in all these areas as well as others like the wounded warriors. It is hoped that the model supervised training program described herein might morph into teams all over the country, providing affordable training and even uniting in a League of Wellness and Motor Behavior Laboratories. The impact of this extended health care model on American health care would be significant.

The prospect of rallying wellness and motor behavior is alluring. We watch every day as people who have been released from conventional care, under our supervision, experience healing. We cannot report that the improvement in their wellness and motor behavior was due of the low-intensity, high-repetition supervised exercise program. Likely attributable to a combination of factors perhaps, as Rediger (*A Medicine of Hope and Possibility* 2015) suggested, the kinesiology team in the LWMB may have managed to add the spark that changed the clients' perceptions of themselves. Nevertheless, I am encouraged that we may have reached a "Tipping Point," (M. Gladwell 2000) where twenty years of "little things can make a big difference." Will our enduring efforts be rewarded? Will people and resources come to such an extended health-care model? James Earl Jones playing radical professional writer Terence Mann in *Field of Dreams*, said to Kevin Costner playing Ray Kinsella on any prospect of returns from the near financial ruin from his sacrificial building of the baseball diamond in his cornfield:

People will come, Ray. They'll come to Iowa for reasons they can't even fathom. They'll turn up your driveway not knowing for sure why they're doing it, and arrive at your door, as innocent as children, longing for the past. "Of course, we won't mind if you look around," you'll say. "It's only twenty dollars per person." And they'll pass over the money without even looking at it. For it is money they have, and peace they lack. (Kinsella 1988)

There's a new ball game in town. We see in our lab every day brilliant minds are trapped inside failing bodies—failing because of disuse. I am not willing to wait until the lights go out. We will assume the risk of being evidence driven and continue to make people better. We've developed a team approach to rehabilitation that is not conventional, and it doesn't have to be disruptive. Let's coin a new phrase. Let's create a new industry— Team Kinesiology[SM] (TK). Maybe this time we don't have to wait to be data driven. Maybe we can move forward, encouraged by the stories with evidence. Maybe this time we don't have to create a rigid structure that destroys creativity. In the search for solutions; maybe it's time to recognize as in education, the futility of using standardized methods to measure nonstandard people. After catastrophic disease or injury, you'll go to speech therapy (ST), occupational therapy (OT), physical therapy (PT) then you will find access to TK, where your efforts to improve wellness and motor behavior will find unending support *after everybody else gave up.*

Our current record-holder in the LWMB, Jerry's appreciation and humility was evident in this September 2014 post on Google+:

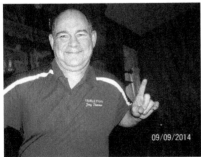 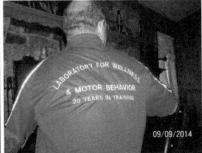

Dr. Priest we started this adventure the second week of July 1994 it seem almost like yesterday since we got to know each other... you introduced me to a machine called a Psycle. Wow how time really flies and the days, weeks, months and years go by. Thanks for making them great and helping me achieve so much. The friendships with you and the helpers and clients has a special place in my heart. I am looking to keep riding the Psycle as long as I can. (Thornton 2014)

Jerry's downstream medical costs were evidently near zero. I can't claim Jerry's distinguished degree of wellness, but then I haven't logged two thousand five hundred complete cardiovascular workouts like he has. We are drug- and supplement-free except for Jerry's multivitamins, and the only side effects of our program are the benefits of habitual exercise. Put a number on that.

Don Larson pitched a perfect game for the New York Yankees in the fifth game of the 1956 World Series against the

Brooklyn Dodgers. Analysis of the pitch selection, the speed and placement would reveal little because of the ever-changing variables in the game. Trying to predetermine an exercise treatment protocol for disease and disability is like trying to predetermine the selection of pitches, speed, and placement prior to the game.

Team Kinesiology^{SM} has a chance—selfless managers who can talk the talk and veteran players who can walk the walk. We have open communication and explicit support of each other. When one talks, everybody listens. Everyone has importance and a respected opinion. We value each other as members of a family—for what we know and what we represent, not by what we can find on the iPhone. We have genuine conversations with no motive. We have no private or whispered conversations, no shouts of shallow-minded Internet answers, interrupting the search for solutions. The individual value to the team is not determined by the batting average, which doesn't tell the whole story—the sacrifice bunts in which the player gives up his at bat for the betterment of the team, and the intentional walks where the opponent pitches around you. We still play for the love of the game, and we want to knock this one out of the park.

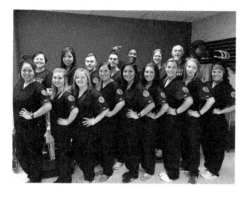

As a health-care industry, it's late in the game and we're losing. Let's bring in our closer to add the spark that starts the rally. Either way, the game will soon be over. I stood in awe at the foot of the Michelangelo's sixteenth-century marble statue of David. The solutions for Dignity 'n Retirement may be as much artistic, spiritual, and evidential as scientific. I have heard the sound of change coming. You heard it too didn't you?

References

Adelman, G., S. G. Rane, and K. F. Villa. 2013. "The Cost Burden of Multiple Sclerosis in the United States: a Systematic Review of the Literature." *Journal of Medical Economics* 16 (5): 639-647.

American College of Sports Medicine. 2009. *ACSM's Exercise is Medicine: A Clinician's Guide to Exercise Prescription.* Philadelphia: Wolters Kluwer and Lippincott Williams & Wilkins.

———. 2014. *ACSM's Guidelines for Exercise Testing and Prescription.* Edited by L. S. Pescatello. Philadelphia, PA: Wolters Kluwer Health/Lippincott Williams & Wilkins.

American Psychological Association. 2009. "Sedentary Lives Can be Deadly: Physical Inactivity Poses Greatest Health Risk to Americans, Expert Says." *ScienceDaily*, August 10. www.sciencedaily.com/releases/2009/08/090810024825. htm.

Anderson, Greg. 2001. *The Triumphant Patient.* Lincoln, NE: iUniverse.com, Inc.

Athritis Foundation. 2016. Mission and Vision. Accessed March 3, 2016. http://www.arthritis.org/about-us/mission-vision.php.

Balkenbush, C., and J. Priest. 2003. "Electromyographic Activity in the Legs of an Individual with Spinal Dysgenesis During Passive Leg Cycling." *Medicine and Science in Sports and Exercise* 35 (5).

Balkenbush, C., M. Sanderford, and J. Priest. 2005. "Effect of Arm-Powered Passive Leg Cycling on Heart Rate Variability in Spinal Cord Injured Individuals." *Medicine and Science in Sports and Exercise* 37 (5).

Banarto, A. E., M. B. McClellen, C. R. Kagay, and A. M. Garber. 2004. Trends in Inpatient Treatment Intensity Among Medicare Beneficiaries at the End of Life." *Health Services Resources* 39 (2): 363-75.

Bauman, A. E., J. F. Sallis, D. A. Dzewaltowski, and N. Owen. 2002. "Toward a Better Understanding of the Influences on Physical Activity: the Role of Determinants, Correlates, Causal Variables, Mediators, Moderators, and Confounders." *American Journal of Preventive Medicine.* 23 (2 Suppl): 5-14.

Bell, Michael. 2013. *Why 5% of Patients Create 50% of Health Care Costs.* Jan. 10. http://www.forbes.com/sites/michaelbell/2013/01/10/why-5-of-patients-create-50-of-health-care-costs/.

Benson, Herbert. 1975. *The Relaxation Response*. New York, NY: William Morrow and Company, Inc.

Bergdahl, Michael. 2006. *The Ten Rules of Sam Walton: Success Secrets for Remarkable Results*. Hoboken, NJ: John Wiley & Sons, Inc.

Berryman, J. 1992. "Exercise and the Medical Tradition from Hippocrates through Antebellum Ameria: A Review Essay." *In Sport and Exercise Science: Essays in the History of Sports Medicine*, by J. Berryman and R.J. Park, 1-56. Urbana and Chicago: University of Illinois.

Bill, Blake. 2015. Google+. September 18. https://plus.google.com/u/0/communities/112013677417890656684.

———. 2015. *Google+*. October 9. https://plus.google.com/u/0/communities/112013677417890656684.

Blankenship, M. and J. Priest. 2000. "Paraplegic Training." *Fitness Management* 16 (2): 46-47.

Blevins, Dustin. 2015. Google+. Jan. 30. https://plus.google.com/u/1/101704876910390668395/posts/LZkaz3ph4H8?cfem=1.

Bollinger, Sara. 2015. Google+. July 29. https://plus.google.com/communities/112013677417890656684?cfem=1.

Boody, Travis. 2015. Google+. Apr 3. https://plus.google.com/u/1/communities/112013677417890656684.

BrainandSpinalCord.org. 2015. *How Many People are Affected by Spinal Cord Injury (SCI)?* July 27. http://www.brain-andspinalcord.org/spinal-cord-injury/prognosis/how-many-people-affected-by-spinal-cord-injury.html.

Caruso, Ty. 2015. Google+. Feb 26. https://plus.google.com/u/1/communities/112013677417890656684?c fem=1.

Centers for Disease Control and Prevention. 1998. *Office Visits to Orthopedic Surgeons.* October 7. Accessed Jan. 7, 2016. http://www.cdc.gov/nchs/pressroom/98facts/ortho.htm.

————. 2014. *Arthritis.* Nov. 12. Accessed Aug. 31, 2015. http://www.cdc.gov/arthritis/.

————. 2015. *Stroke Facts.* March 24. Accessed July 27, 2015. http://www.cdc.gov/stroke/facts.htm.

————. 2015. July 27. http://www.cdc.gov/ncbddd/cp/data.html.

CerebralPalsy.org. 2015. the Ultimate Resource for Everything Cerebral Palsy. July 27. http://cerebralpalsy.org/about-cerebral-palsy/prevalence-and-incidence/.

Chavez, Sammie, interview by J. W. Priest. 2016. Student-intern (January 20).

Christopher & Dana Reeve Foundation. 2016. Today's care. Tomorrow's Cure. Accessed March 1, 2016. http://

www.christopherreeve.org/site/c.mtKZKgMWKw-G/b.5184189/k.5587/Paralysis_Facts__Figures.htm.

Cisneros, Elizabeth. 2015. Google+. October 2.

———. 2015. Google+. October 22. https://plus.google.com/u/0/communities/112013677417890656684.

Clark, Jamie. 2015. Google+. October 23. https://plus.google.com/u/0/communities/112013677417890656684.

Cooper, Kenneth. 1968. *Aerobics.* New York: M. Evans and Co. and Bantam Books.

———. 1982. *The Aerobics Program for Total Well-Being.* Toronto, New York, London, Sydney, and Auckland: Bantam Books.

———. 1985. *Running Without Fear.* Toronto, New York, London, Sydney, and Auckland: Bantam Books.

Cruwys, T., S. A. Haslam, and G. A. Dingle. 2014. "The New Group Therapy." *Scientific American Mind: Behavior, Brain Science, Insights* Sept/Oct: 61-63.

Cumby, Casey, interview by J. W. Priest. 2015. Dad (Jan 21).

Cumby, Misty, interview by J. W. Priest. 2015. Mom (Feb 11).

Dawes, Doyle. 2015. Google+. Apr 2. https://plus.google.com/u/1/communities/112013677417890656684.

DeVivo, M. J., Yuing Chen, S. T. Mennemeyer, and A. Deutsch. 2011. "Costs of Care Following Spinal Cord Injury." *Spinal Cord Injury Rehabilitation* 16 (4): 1-9.

Dodd, K. J., N. F. Taylor, and D. L. Damiano. 2002. "A Systematic Review of the Effectiveness of Strength-Training Programs for People with Cerebral Palsy." *Archives of Physical Medicine and Rehabilitation* 83 (8): 1157-1164.

Edge, Chris. 2015. Google+. September 25. https://plus.google.com/u/0/communities/112013677417890656684.

Einstein, Albert. 1950. *Out of My Later Years.* New York: Philosophical Library.

————. 1952. "Jungkaufmann." *Schweizerischer Kaufmaennischer Verein, Jugendbund*, Feb 29.

————. 1954. "On Classic Literature." In *Ideas and Opinions by Albert Einstein*, by Albert

Einstein, edited by Carl Seelig, translated by Sonja Bargmann, 64-65. Avenel, NJ: Wings Books.

Ellis, Alyne. 2011. "Prime Time Focus." *AARP: The Magazine*, June 8.

Ferguson, J., and J. Priest. 2000. "Electromyographic Responses in a C7 Tetraplegic During Passive Leg Cycling." *Medicine and Science in Sports and Exercise* 32 (5).

Ferguson, Thomas, interview by J. W. Priest. 2015. Student-Intern (Feb 9).

Finley, Lauren. 2015. Google+. July 1. https://plus.google.com/communities/112013677417890656684.

Foege, William H. 1985. "Public Health and Preventive Medicine." *Journal of the American Medical Association*.

Frenkel, H.S. 1902. *The Treatment of Tabetic Ataxia by Means of Systematic Exercises*. Philadelphia: P. Blakiston's Son & Co.

Fulfer, Sarah, interview by J. W. Priest. 2015. LWMB Supervisor (Mar 30).

Garber, C. E., B. Blissmer, M. R. Deschenes, et al. 2011. "American College of Sports Medicine Position Stand; Quantity and Quality of Exercise for Developing and Maintaining Cardiorespiratory, Musculoskeletal, and Neuromotor Fitness in Apparently Healthy Adults." *Medicine and Science in Sports and Exercise* 43 (7): 1334-1359.

Gardner, R., and J. Priest. 2002. "Effects of Repetitive Movement on the Electromyographic Response of the Triceps in a C5 Tetraplegic." *Medicine and Science in Sports and Exercise* 33 (5).

Gerber, E. 1971. *Innovators and Institutions in Physical Education*. Philadelphia: Lea and Febiger.

Gladwell, Malcolm. 2000. *Tipping Point: How Little Things Can Make a Big Difference.* New York and Boston: Little, Brown and Company.

———. 2005. *Blink: The Power of Thinking Without Thinking.* New York and Boston: Little, Brown and Company.

———. 2008. *Outliers: The Story of Success.* New York, Boston, and London: Little, Brown and Company.

Godfrey, Mike, interview by J. W. Priest. 2015. Client (Jan 9).

Godwin, K. M., J. Wasserman, and S. K. Ostwald. 2011. "Cost Associated with Stroke: Outpatient Rehabilitative Services and Medication." *Topics in Stroke Rehabilitation* 18 Suppl 1: 676-684.

Gold, Sunny Sea. 2014. "How to Be a Better Time Manager." *Scientific American Mind: Behavior, Brain Science, Insights* Sept/Oct: 14.

Grandin, Temple, interview by Lois Parshley. 2015. On How to Raise Resilient Animals (July).

Grant, Meg. 2015, Feb/Mar. "What I Know Now: Valerie Harper." *AARP: The Magazine* 14-17.

Gross, Kurt, interview by J. W. Priest. 2016. Former Client (Jan 27).

Hallal, P. C., L. B. Andersen, F. C. Bull, R. Gothold, W. Haskell, and U. Ekelund. 2012. "Global Physical Activity Level:

Surveillance Progress, Pitfalls, and Progress." *Lancet* 380: 237-257.

Harvey, A., J. Robin, M. E. Morris, H. K. Graham, and R. Baker. 2008. "A Systematic Review of Measures of Activity Limitation for Children with Cerebral Palsy." *Developmental Medicine and Child Neurology* 50 (3): 190-198.

Healthwise Staff. 2014. "Spinal Cord Injury: Autonomic Dysreflexia". WebMD. Accessed March 12. http://www. webmd.com/hypertension-high-blood-pressure/tc/spi-nal-cord-injury-autonomic-dysreflexia-topic-overview.

Hernandez, Jaimie. 2015. Google+. October 16. https://plus. google.com/u/0/communities/112013677417890656684.

Hite, Ashley. 2015. Discussion Board. June 9. https://black-boardlearn.tarleton.edu/webapps/discussionboard/do/message?forum_id=_72591_1&layer=forum&nav=dis-cussion_board_entry&action=collect_for_stu_review_forward&origRequestId=D7C55D22650048E76D-15B25ADC9A554B_1433954300767&conf_id=_46803_1&user_id=_1.

Holmes, Oliver Wendell. 1858. The Deacon's Masterpiece or The Wonderful "One Hoss Shay": A Logical Story. Legal Language. Feb 2. https://www.legallanguage.com/resources/poems/onehossshay/.

Hooper, Jaycie. 2015. Discussion Board. June 5. https://black-boardlearn.tarleton.edu/webapps/discussionboard/do/

message?forum_id=_72591_1&layer=forum&nav=dis-cussion_board_entry&action=collect_for_stu_review_forward&origRequestId=F0435EE90380B7D4B-3F7A08128AB5F6D_1433768890002&conf_id=_46803_1&user_id=_8.

International Brain Injury Association, Interview with Ronald Savage, Ed.D., http://www.internationalbrain.org/articles/-interview-with-ron-savage-edd/ April 9, 2013, accessed February 20, 2016.

Ivanyi, B., M. Schoenmakers, N. van Veen, K. Maathuis, F. Nollet, and M. Nederhand. 2014. "The Effects of Orthoses, Footwear, and Walking Aids on the Walking Ability of Children and Adolescents with Spina Bifida: A Systematic Review Using International Classification of Functioning, Disability and Health for Children and Youth (ICF-CY)." *Prosthetics and Orthotics International* 39(6):437-43.

Jackson, Trentin, interview by J. W. Priest. 2015. Student-Intern (Apr 3).

Johnson, Chelsea, interview by J. W. Priest. 2014. Client (Nov 14).

Kancherla, V.D., Amendah, S. Grosse, M. Yeargin-Allsopp, and B. Van Naarden. 2012. "Medical Expenditures Attributable to Cerebral Palsy and Intellectual Disability Among Medicaid-enrolled Children." *Research in Developmental Disabilities* 33(3): 832-40.

Kinsella, W.P. 1988. Field of Dreams. Directed by Phil Alden Robinson. http://www.imsdb.com/scripts/Field-of-Dreams.html.

Kohutek, Alysha. 2015. Student-Intern. Mar 17. https://plus.google.com/communities/112013677417890656684?fd=1.

Krassioukov, A. 2012. "Autonomic Dysreflexia: Current Evidence Related to Unstable Arterial Blood Pressure Control Among Athletes with Spinal Cord Injury." *Clinical Journal of Sports Medicine* 22 (1): 39-45.

Kruse, M., S. Michelsen, E. Flachs, H. Bronnum-Hansen, M. Medsen, P. Uldall. 2009. "Lifetime Costs of Cerebral Palsy." *Developmental Medicine and Child Neurology* 51(8):622-8.

Leu, Christopher, interview by J. W. Priest. 2016. President Texas Health Harris Methodist Hospital (Feb. 19).

Love, Robert, ed. 2015, Feb/Mar. "Costly Couch Potatoes." *AARP: The Magazine* 4.

Maianu, Marius. 2015. "CooperAerobics – Cooper Aerobics – Your VO2 Max and Why You Should Know That Number". CooperAerobics. Feb 17. http://cooperaerobics.com/Health-Tips/Prevention-Plus/Benefits-of-Knowing-Your-VO2-Max.aspx#.VONaS4Kl2YA.email.

Mamach, Victoria. interview by J. W. Priest. 2015. Student/Intern (August 25).

———. 2015. Google+. October 9. https://plus.google. com/u/0/communities/112013677417890656684.

Manigold, Blaine, interview by J. W. Priest. 2015. Client (Mar 26).

Mason, Fred. 2008. "R. Tate McKenzie's Medical Work and Early Exercise Therapies for People with Disabilities." *Sport History Review* 39: 45-70.

Mathews, Julia. 2015. Google+. Jan. 29. https://plus.google. com/u/1/104822676331986643498/posts?cfem=1.

Mauldin, Bailee. 2015. Google+. Feb. 6. https://plus.google. com/u/1/communities/112013677417890656684/s/ incredible?cfem=1.

———. 2015. Google+. Feb 20. https://plus.google.com/u/1/ communities/112013677417890656684?cfem=1.

———. 2015. Google+. Aug 28. https://plus.google.com/ communities/112013677417890656684?cfem=1.

———. 2015. Google+. October 10. https://plus.google. com/u/0/communities/112013677417890656684.

Mazur, J. M. 2004. "Efficacy of Bracing the Lower Limbs and Ambulation Training in Children with Myelomeningocele." *Developmental Medicine and Child Neurology* 46: 352-356.

McArdle, W. D., F. I. Katch, and V. L. Katch. 2007. *Exercise Physiology: Energy, Nutrition, and Human Performance.* 6. Philadelphia: Lippincott Williams and Wilkins.

McKenzie, R. Tate. 1894. "The Therapeutic Uses of Exercise." *Montreal Medical Journal* 560-572.

———. 1909. *Exercise in Education and Medicine.* Philadelphia/London: W.B. Saunders Co.

———. 1915. "Treatment of Convalenscent Soldies by Physical Means." *American Physical Education Review* 31-70.

———. 1917. "Treatment of Convalescent Soldiers by Physical Means." *American Physical Education Review* 33-36.

———. 1918. "Reclaiming the Maimed at War." *New York Medical Journal* 556.

———. 1918. *Reclaiming the Maimed: A Handbook of Physical Therapy.* New York: McMillan.Mellen Center for Multiple Sclerosis, Cleveland Clinic. 2014. WebMD, LLC. National Multiple Sclerosis Society. October 25. Accessed October 31, 2015. http://www.webmd.com/multiple-sclerosis/guide/multiple-sclerosis-physical-therapy.

Moeller, Phillip. 2011. "Senior Villages Take Root as Movement Matures." *U. S. News and World Report: Money,* January 28. Accessed December 10, 2015. http://money.usnews.com/money/blogs/the-best-life/2011/01/28/senior-villages-take-root-as-movement-matures.

Moore, Jeffery, interview by J. W. Priest. 2015. Client (October 26).

National Center for Chronic Disease Prevention and Health Promotion. 2013. *The State of Aging and Health in America 2013*. Atlanta, GA: US Department of Health and Human Services.

National Multiple Sclerosis Society. 2015. MS Prevalence. June 17. Accessed July 27, 2015. http://www.nationalms-society.org/About-the-Society/MS-Prevalence.

———. 2016. "Raise Awareness". National Multiple Sclerosis Society. Accessed March 2, 2016. http://www.nationalms-society.org/Get-Involved/Raise-Awareness.

National Stroke Association. 2016. Hope After Stroke. Accessed March 1, 2016. http://www.stroke.org/.

Nelson, Miriam E. 2012. "Staying Active and Social Prolongs Life Even After 75." Health and Nutrition Letter, Dec.

Office of Communications and Public Liaison (NIH). 2004. Stroke: Hope Through Research. July. http://www.ninds.nih.gov/disorders/stroke/stroke.htm.

Ogunola, Ebun. 2015. Google+. Jan. 30. https://plus.google.com/u/1/116594800224539564285/posts?cfem=1.

Park, R. 2008. "Setting the Scene - Bridging the Gap between Knowledge and Practice: When Americans Really Built Programmes to Foster Healthy Lifestyles." *The International Journal of the History of Sport* 1427-52.

Pratt, Rickie, interview by J. W. Priest. 2015. Client (Mar 17).

Priest, J, D. Hagan, S. Simpson, and R. Jennings. 1996. "Improved Exercise Capacity of Paraplegics Following Eight Weeks of Unassisted Leg Cycle Training." *Medicine and Science in Sports and Exercise* 28 (5).

Pugh, J. 1794. *Physiological, theoretical and practical treatise on the utility of the science of muscular motion for restoring the power of the limbs.* London: Dilly.

Ransom, Cliff, ed. 2015. "Dare to Dream Big." *Popular Science* 6.

Rediger, Jeffrey. 2015. "A Medicine of Hope and Possibility." TEDxNewBedford. New Bedford, MA, Nov 6. Accessed Jan 14, 2016. https://www.youtube.com/watch?v=8mjVHIB0FhI.

Rheinlaender, Colton. 2015. Google+. Jan. 30. https://plus.google.com/u/1/communities/112013677417890656684/s/colton?cfem=1.

Riebe, D. A., B. A. Franklin, P. D. Thompson, C. E. Garber, G. P. Whitfield, M. Magal, and L. S. Pescatello. 2015. "Updating ACSM's Recommentation for Exercise Preparticipation Health Screening." *Medicine and Science in Sports and Exercise* 47 (11): 2476.

Rizzuto, D., N. Orsini, C. Qiu, H. Wang, and L. Fratiglioni. 2012. "Lifestyle, Social Factors, and Survival After Age 75: Population Based Study." *British Medical Journal* 345:e5568.

Robinson, Ken. 2006. "Do Schools Kill Creativity?" TEDtalks: Ideas Worth Sharing. Monterey, CA, Feb. Accessed Jan 15, 2016. http://www.ted.com/talks/ken_robinson_says_schools_kill_creativity.

Robinson, Ken. 2013. "How to Escape Education's Death Valley." TEDtalks: Ideas Worth Sharing. April. Accessed Jan 13, 2016. https://www.youtube.com/watch?v=wX78iKhInsc.

Rogers, Naomi. 1996. *Dirt and Disease: Polio Before FDR.* New Bunswick, New Jersey: Rutgers.

Rossman, Martin L. 2000. *Guided Imagery for Self-Healing.* Novato, CA: H.J. Kramer; a joint venture with New World Library.

Sallis, Robert E. 2009. "Foreword in Exercise is Medicine™." *In ACSM's Exercise is Medicine™: A Clinician's Guide to Exercise Prescription,* by Steven Jonas, vii. Philadelphia: Wolters Kluwer Health and Lippincott Williams & Wilkins.

Sherrill, Claudine. 1993. *Adapted Physical Activity, Recreation and Sport.* Madison, WI, Dubuque, IO, Indianapolis, IN, Melbourne, Australia, Oxford, England: Brown & Benchmark Publishers.

Siedel, Edward. 2013. "The Greatest Retirement Crisis In American History." *Forbes,* March 20.

Simpson, S. and J. Priest. 2005. "Conditioning in Injured and Disabled Populations." *Strength and Conditioning Journal* 27 (6).

Skaggs, William. 2014. "New Neurons for New Memories." *Scientific American Mind: Behavior, Brain Science, Insights*, Sept/Oct: 49-53.

Smith, Randy, interview by J. W. Priest. 2015. Client (Jan. 15).

Snodgrass, Chandler. 2015. Google+. October 23. https://plus.google.com/u/0/communities/112013677417890656684.

Sohm, Irene, interview by J. W. Priest. 2015. Client (Feb 5).

Spina Bifida Association. 2015. Educators: Health Information Sheets. Accessed March 2, 2016. http://spinabifidaassociation.org/educators/.

Spitzer, Courtney. 2015. Google+. July 29. https://plus.google.com/communities/112013677417890656684.

Spitzer, Courtney, interview by Andrew Wolfe. 2015. Student-Intern (July 6).

Spitzer, Courtney, interview by J. W. Priest. 2015. Student-Intern (Aug 3).

Stahl, J. E., M. L. Dossett, A. S. LaJoie, J. W. Denninger, D. H. Mehta, R. Goldman, G. L. Fricchione, and H. Benson. 2015. "Relaxation Response and Resiliency Training and Its Effect on Healtcare Resource Utilization." *PLoS One* 10 (10): e0140212.

Stock, Emily. 2015. Google+. Aug 28. https://plus.google.com/communities/112013677417890656684?cfem=1.

————. 2015. Google+. October 15. https://plus.google.com/communities/112013677417890656684?cfem=1.

Sutherland, Neal, interview by J. W. Priest. 2015. Physician (Sept. 21).

Swydan, Paul, ed. n.d. The Hardball Times. Accessed Jan. 1, 2016. http://www.hardballtimes.com/tht-live/30000-day-versary-the-greatest-world-series-comeback/#comments.

Thomas, Lewis. 1979. *The Medusa and the Snail.* New York, NY: The Viking Press.

Thornton, Jerry, interview by J. W. Priest. 2014. Long-time Client (Sept 9).

U.S. Department of Commerce. 2015. "United States Census Bureau." Newsroom. June 25. Accessed Jan 22, 2016. http://www.census.gov/newsroom/press-releases/2015/cb15-113.html.

"U.S. News and World Report". 2015. U.S. News and World Report. Edited by Kerry Dyer. U.S. News & World Report, LLC. Sept. 23. http://www.usnews.com/info/features/about-usnews.

UAB/Lakeshore Research Collaboration. 2015. "Exercise for Individuals with Spina Bifilda: NCHPAD – Building Healthy Inclusive Communities." National Center on Health, Physical Activity, and Disability (NCHPAD). October 31. http://www.nchpad.org/239/1561/Exercises~for~Individuals~with~Spina~Bifida.

United Cerebral Palsy. 2015. Life Without Limits for People with Disabilities. Accessed March 2, 2016. http://ucp. org/.

University of Alabama. 2006. UAB Model SCI System. June. http://www.spinalcord.uab.edu/show.asp?durki=21446.

van der Woude, L. H., S. de Groot, K. Postema, J. B. Bussmann, T. W. Janssen, and M. W. Post ALLRISC. 2013. "Active LifestyLe Rehabilitation Interventions in Aging Spinal Cord Injury (ALLRISC): a Multicentre Research Program." *Disability Rehabilitation* 35 (13): 1097-1103.

Vankoski, S. J., C. Moore, K. D. Statler, et al. 1997. "The Influence of Forearm Crutches on Pelvic and Hip Kinematics in Children with Myelomeningocele: Don't Throw Away the Crutches." *Developmental Medicine and Child Neurology* 39: 614-619.

WebMD. 2015. Stroke Health Center. Oct. 1. http://www. webmd.com/stroke/tc/stroke-rehabilitation-what-to-ex-pect-after-a-stroke?page=2.

Willoughby, D. S., J. Priest, and M. Nelson. 2002. "Expression of the Stress Proteins, Ubiquitin, and HSP-72, and Myofibrillar Protein Content After Passive Leg Cycling in Persons with Spinal Cord Injury." *Archives of Physical Medicine and Rehabilitation* 83: 649-654.

Willoughby, D. S., J. Priest, and R. Jennings. 2000. "Myosin Heavy-Chain Isoform and Ubiquitin Protease mRNA After Passive Leg Cycling in Persons with Spinal Cord

Injury." *Archives of Physical Medicine and Rehabilitation* 81: 157-163.

Wolfe, Andy, interview by J. W. Priest. 2015. Former NCAA baseball player (Dec. 12).

World Health Organization. 2002. Media Center. April 4. http://www.who.int/mediacentre/news/releases/release 23/en/.

About the Author

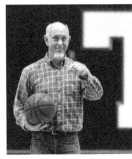

Born in Coleman County, Texas, Joe W. Priest grew up in the farming community of Olton, Texas where he participated in band and athletics. He attended Sul Ross State University where he was a

Author Photo by Kurt Mogonye, Tarleton State University, Creative Services Coordinator

quarterback on the NAIA football team. There he completed his BS degree and his master's degree in biology. He coached and taught biology for ten years before returning to study at Texas A&M-Commerce, where he completed his EdD degree in 1983. He spent eight years in corporate fitness prior to beginning twenty-five years as a professor at Tarleton State University. In the Department of Kinesiology, he teaches exercise physiology, kinesiology, exercise electrocardiography, and biomechanics. His Laboratory for Wellness and Motor Behavior has provided access to the benefits of exercise for individuals who have various degrees of paralysis from injury or disease.

CPSIA information can be obtained
at www.ICGtesting.com
Printed in the USA
FSOW04n2140240317
32319FS